A
NEW LOOK
Into the
OLD BOOK

Ruth Lascelle

A
NEW LOOK
Into the
OLD BOOK

A New Look Into the Bible
to
Be in Health

by
Ruth Specter Lascelle

ℬ

Bedrock Publishing
Arlington, Washington

Library of Congress Cataloging-in-Publication Data
Lascelle, Ruth Specter. (Part 1) *A New Look Into the Old Book*; (Part 2) *To Be in Health* / Ruth Specter Lascelle. Editor, Duane Bagaas. Associate Editor, Wuffy Evans. Illustrated with graphics. Bibliography. General Index.
(Part 1): *A New Look Into the Old Book:* 1. Strange Titles, 2. Scientific Development, 3. Notes in My Bible, 4. How to Study the Bible, 5. Answers to some misunderstood questions.
(Part 2): *Be in Health.* 1. Laughter/Emotions, 2. Phobias, 3. Diet/Gluttony, 6. Fasting, 7. Apostle Paul's thorn in the flesh.

Library of Congress Catalog Card Number: 98-071625
ISBN 0-9654519-0-9

Cover design by Bedrock Publishing

Printed in the United States of America
by
Gorham Printing
Rochester, Washington

Dedicated to all those who love the Word of God and who follow its instructions for health in spirit, soul and body.

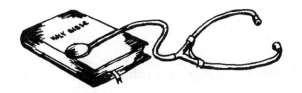

Books by Ruth Specter Lascelle

A Dwelling Place for God (revised and enlarged edition)
A New Look Into the Old Book: To Be in Health
God's Calendar of Prophetic Events: "Leviticus Twenty-Three"
Hanukkah and Christmas
How Shall They Hear? (With Hyman Israel Specter)
Jewish Faith and The New Covenant
Jewish Love for a Gentile: "Story of The Lascelles"
My Jewish People
New Covenant Passover Haggadah: "Remembering The Exodus of Deliverance"
On What Day Did Christ Die? "The Last Week of Christ"
Pictures of Messiah in The Holy Scriptures
That They Might be Saved: "Eight Lessons in Jewish Evangelism"
The Global Harvest
The Passover Feast
Two Loaves—One Bread: "Jew and Gentile in the Church"
We Have a Great High Priest: "A Brief Study of The Book of Hebrews"

No longer in print:
   Mission to Haiti
   Sent Forth by God
   The Bud and The Flower of Judaism

AUTHOR'S PREFACE

Ever since I learned of Corrie ten Boom's declaration: *"I got a new look at the Old Book,"* I wanted that same experience.

Some of the writing which I have included here is taken from others who found special meanings in the Scriptures. While studying God's Word, I was enabled by the Holy Spirit to find new truths which are inserted into this volume. It is hoped that these findings will help the reader also to "take a new look into the Old Book."

The first section of Part 1 comprise articles about the Bible itself; the last section is concerning answers to Bible questions most often misunderstood. This by no means covers the subjects entirely. Some of these items appear at length in other books I have written. Here, it is a concentrated study to inspire the readers toward further research.

It is hoped that Section 5 of Part 1, which includes a system of Bible Study, will help the reader in studying God's wonderful Word.

I cannot ignore the fact that God chose the *Jewish people* to write His Word. Therefore, to understand the Bible we should investigate its *Hebraic* setting. I would like to stress the importance of looking into the Scriptures with the **Jewish background in mind**. This will make the "old book" more like the *new book* that it is!

> The theologian Thomas F. Torrance has remarked challengingly: "How can we see Jesus the Jew from Bethlehem, Nazareth and Jerusalem, without the use of *Jewish* eyes? ... I was looking through lenses of Gentile spectacles which distorted what was there, so that I had to learn to take off the spectacles I did not even know I was wearing."[1]

To illustrate one of the reasons, other than the advice of Corrie ten Boom, the following experience shows why I was impressed to write this book:

One of the first evangelistic efforts which the Lord honored me to conduct was in the year 1955 at Broadway Tabernacle located in Vancouver, British Columbia, Canada where Dr. E. T. Robinson was Pastor. One night I gave a message on "The Tabernacle of Moses," emphasizing the article of furniture in the Holy of Holies named "The Ark of the Covenant." When I declared that the broken law inside the Ark of the Covenant was covered over by the sacrificial blood on the Mercy Seat, the power of God by the Holy Spirit was poured out upon

---

[1] *The Witness of the Jews to God,* edited by D.W. Torrance (Handsel Press, Edinburgh, 1982).

the congregation. All those present were excited to worship our wonderful Lord for some time before I was able to continue with the message.

After the service in the pastor's home, he questioned me: "Where in the Bible did you find that the broken law of God was inside the Ark of the Covenant and covered over by the sacrificial blood on the Mercy Seat"?

I stuttered out that I had heard this from another evangelist who mentioned that outstanding truth from the Tabernacle services and I copied it. When he did, the very same thing took place that happened "tonight": The blessing of God came down upon the people.

Dr. Robinson repeated: "But, Miss Specter, where did you find that *in the Bible*?"

I confessed I didn't find it in the Bible but it must be true if God's blessings accompanied it so as to give His stamp of approval.

Pastor Robinson replied: "You should be certain that what you preach lines up with the Words of God. Be like the Bereans who searched the Scriptures *to see whether these things were so.* The *broken* law was *not* deposited in the Ark of the Covenant, Miss Specter. It was the *unbroken* law that was kept there. A much greater truth is found in this than that the *broken* law was inside the Ark, etc."

From that day–though preachers and writers have presented what they feel is truth which is accompanied by a great blessing–I always remember what Dr. Robinson advised me. I search through the Scriptures to see whether "these things are so." By doing this I have discovered many precious "jewels," truths which are shared with God's people to whom I have had the privilege to minister!

Especially in Section 3 of "A New Look Into the Old Book," I am giving a few truths (out of many more) which the Holy Spirit has enlightened to my heart. It is my prayer that the Holy Spirit will use this entire volume to show w*hat the Bible says* and will help the readers to *take a new look into the old book.*

Part Two of this book is the addition entitled "Be in Health" which was to be printed as a separate volume. This seemed appropriate to combine with "A New Look Into the Old Book" since Health is found in the Word of God.

Table of Contents

Part 1 – A New Look Into the Old Book 1
Section 1: Books of the Bible 1
   The Books of the Bible 1
   Bible University 3
Section 2: Articles About the Bible 5
   The Bible 5
   The Book 5
   The Textbook Says: ...... But God Says: 6
   Bibles With Strange Titles 7
   The Bible is Full of Mistakes 10
   Great Books 11
   Facts No One Can Dodge 12
   The Bible Scientifically Accurate 18
   The Scriptures Divinely Inspired 19
   Jesus and the Scriptures 20
   Messiah and the Old Testament 20
   The Bible has 8,810 Promises 21
   Is That in the Bible? 24
   A Beautiful Tribute to the Bible 28
   The Holy Bible for Girls and Boys 29
   Bible Acrostic 31
   Questions Answered by Ernest S. Williams 31
   "Skin of Your Teeth" is Real 32
   General Science of the Book of Job 33
   Scientific Facts Established 34
   The Inspiration of the Scriptures Scientifically
      Demonstrated.. 34
   The Hairs of Your Head are Numbered 36
   Emotional Drunkards 37
   Proverbs 38
   The Song of Degrees 39

Section 3: Inspirational Truths 41
    In the Beginning 41
    God Created the Alphabet 42
    God Reveals His Name to Moses 44
    The Dream 46
Section 4: Answers to Some Misunderstood
    Questions 47
    Cain's Wife–Where did He Get Her? 47
    Train up a Child (A misunderstood statement in
      the Bible.) 49
    Rapture or Destruction, Which? 50
    Can We Command God? 52
    Did God Give Israel Power to get Wealth? 52
Section 5: How to Study the Bible 53
    Bible Study 53
    In Studying Your Bible Look for the Flags 54
Section 6: Notes in My Bible 57
    The Bible 57
    Be Ye Doers of the Word (James 1:22) 58
    Bible Study 58
    Read the Bible 59
    The Bible Speaks 61
    The Word of God in the 119th Psalm 62
    Verse Numbering in the Bible 63
    Seven Deadly Sins 67
    Growing Old 67
    The People of the Book 68
    Importance of "Know-How" 68
    Teaching Jewish Children 69
    Plurality of "Elohim" 70
    Plurality and Unity 71
    The Man, Moses 71
    Edom (Esau)–Mount Sier 72
    Discover the Holy Place 73
    Isaiah 53 in Jewish Writings 74
    The Key of David 74

Points for Preachers 75
God Did Not Call Me 75
Vinegar and Water 80
Milk and Honey 81
Part 2 – Be In Health 83
Section 1: Healing in the Bible 84
God Created the Spirit, Soul and Body 84
God Promised Healing to Israel 85
Lord of Health 87
Healing is 88
Be Strong 89
Healing of the Nations 91
How to Stay Healthy 91
How Thought Controls Well-Being 92
Discouragement, the Devil's Tool 93
Effect of Thought in Health and the Body 94
Good Health Department 95
Food From the Bible 96
Healing in the Atonement 97
Prayer for a Sick One 98
Section 2: The Tongue 99
Three Diseases of the Tongue 99
Healing by the Tongue 100
What the Tongue Can Do 103
The Kind and Tender Word 103
Sin of the Tongue 104
The Sin of Backbiting 106
The Sin of Spiritual Cannibalism 108
The Backbiter and His Doom 110
Slander, a Dangerous Weapon 113
Stick Out Your Tongue 114
The Power of the Tongue 116
Talkativeness 117
The Tongue–Good and Bad 120
The Vice of the Mote Hunter 121
Minced Oaths 122

George Washington's View on Profanity............ 123

Section 3: Healing by Laughter 124
He Who Laughs–Lasts 124
Lighten up—Laugh Your Way to Good Health.. 125
Learn to Laugh 126
Healing Power of Laughter 127
Laughter and Fitness 127
Feel Funny, Feel Good 128

Section 4: Related Items on Health 129
The Elderly 129
Go Ahead, Cry Your Eyes Out 130
Hugging is Healthy 130
The Brain 131
Mental Malady 132
Strange Fears of the Mind 132
Remedy to Eliminate Phobias 134

Section 5: Healing Through Diet 135
The Cook or the Book, Which? 135
Heavenly Menu 136
Eating to the Glory of God 136
Calorie Counter's Prayer 142

Section 6: Fasting 143
Is Fasting for Today? 143
Fasting for Health and Healing 146
Food for Thought 147
Gluttony 149
It's Such a Small Sin, Lord 149
The Sin We do not Talk About 151

Section 7: Paul's Thorn in the Flesh 155

Bibliography 160

General Index 161

Part 1

A New Look Into the Old Book

The Books of the Bible

The books of the Bible were written as the result of inspiration and will forever remain mankind's greatest source of inspiration. At the suggestion or under the guidance of the Holy Spirit these men of long ago wrote that which lives and moves again, with informing, uplifting, redeeming power in the hearts and lives of men.

Today, as ever, the Bible occupies an exalted position in literature and of all the books, secular or religious, it has by far the widest distribution over the world. In becoming a religious guide to nearly one-third of the human race, the entire Bible or portions of it have been translated into 400 languages and dialects.

It is interesting to note that the books of the Old and New Testaments of the Holy Bible can be divided into periods and sections so that the Biblical system can be readily grasped. The understanding of these divisions enables one to obtain a fuller comprehension which incites further study. In the following, the poet has very cleverly noted the most important facts of every book of the Bible as well as bringing forth in a very pleasing manner these divisions.

In *GENESIS* the world was made;
In *EXODUS* the march was told;
LEVITICUS contains the law;
In *NUMBERS* are the tribes enrolled.
In *DEUTERONOMY* again
We're urged to keep God's law alone;
Perhaps the oldest writings known.
Brave *JOSHUA* to Canaan leads;
In *JUDGES* oft the Jews rebel;
We read of David's name in *RUTH*,
And *FIRST* and *SECOND KINGS* we read

How bad the Hebrew state became;
In *FIRST* and *SECOND CHRONICLES*
Another history of the same.
In *EZRA* captive Jews return,
And *NEHEMIAH* builds the wall:
Queen *ESTHER* saves her race from death,
These books "historical" we call.
In *JOB* we read of patient faiths;
The *PSALMS* are David's songs of praise;
The *PROVERBS* are to make us wise;
ECCLESIASTES next portrays
How fleeting earthly pleasures are;
The *SONG OF SOLOMON* is all
About the love of Christ. And these
Five books "devotional" we call.
ISAIAH tells of Christ to come,
While *JEREMIAH* tells of woe,
And in his *LAMENTATIONS* mourns
The holy city's overthrow.
EZEKIEL speaks of mysteries,
And *DANIEL* foretells kings of old;
HOSEA calls men to repent,
In *JOEL* blessings are foretold.
AMOS tells of wrath; and Edom
OBADIAH's sent to warn;
While *JONAH* shows that Christ should die
And *MICAH* where He should be born.
In *NAHUM*, Nineveh is seen
In *ZEPHANIAH*, Judah's sins;
In *HAGGAI* the temple built;
ZECHARIAH speaks of Christ,
And *MALACHI*, of John, his sign.
The Prophets number seventeen,
And all the books are thirty-nine.
MATTHEW, MARK and *LUKE* and *JOHN*
Tell what Christ did in every place;
ACTS shows what the apostles did,
And *ROMANS* how we're saved by grace.
CORINTHIANS instructs the Church;
GALATIANS shows of faith alone;
EPHESIANS, true love; and in
PHILIPPIANS God's grace is shown.
COLOSSIANS tells us more of Christ,
And *THESSALONIANS* of the end;
In *TIMOTHY* and *TITUS* both
Are rules for pastors to attend;

PHILEMON Christian friendship shows.
Then *HEBREWS* clearly tells how all
The Jewish laws prefigured Christ.
And these Epistles are by Paul.
JAMES shows that faith by works must live,
And *PETER* urges steadfastness,
While *JOHN* exhorts to Christian love,
For those who have it God will bless.
JUDE shows the end of evil men,
And *REVELATION* tells of heaven.
This ends the whole New Testament
And all the books are twenty-seven.
—Author Unknown

Bible University

by J. S. Eastman

The Bible is similar to a university in that it provides a spiritual education in Christian perspectives.

Genesis is the Medical Department where the embryo of life is developed, the virus of sin produced, the vaccine of faith discovered, and the first anesthesia used.

Exodus is the Department of Sociology on ancient Hebrew culture.

Leviticus is the Law Department, and **Deuteronomy** is a crash course in Law School.

Numbers is a study of God's underground railroad and a geographic survey of the Sinai Peninsula.

Joshua is the West Point where the ROTC's are graduated.

Judges is a study in political science on how to keep a nation morally pure.

Ruth wins the Pulitzer Prize for the best short story on love.

Samuel, **Kings**, and **Chronicles** are the History Department, telling of the rise and fall of the Israeli Empire.

Ezra and **Nehemiah** form the Exploration and Excavation Department of the University.

Esther is a study in dramatics, depicting a nation's deliverance.

Job is the Department of Journalism and offers a study in Philosophy.

Psalms is the Department of Music where instruments are tuned to perfection for praise.

Proverbs is the Chapel on the campus.

Ecclesiastes is human philosophy at its best.

The Song of Solomon is the botanical garden where graduates are united in marriage.

Isaiah to **Malachi** comprise the observatory of astronomy where 16 telescopes are focused on the Bright and Morning Star.

Matthew, Mark, Luke, and **John** are the Editorial Department where students learn about the headlines of the centuries.

Acts is a crash course in church history.

Romans is the Department of Archives in Christian Theology.

Corinthians is a course in apologetics.

Galatians is a simulated court trial where two attorneys, Law and Grace, argue it out.

Ephesians and **Philippians** are a course in design and engineering for blueprinting character and conduct.

Colossians gives us an interview with the President of the University, His pre-eminence is everywhere.

Thessalonians is a course in etiquette, on how to greet the King when He returns.

Timothy is a minister's seminar in the Department of Divinity.

Titus is a beauty course on divine cosmetics.

Philemon is a demonstration course on public relations and psychology.

Hebrews is a course on photography, capturing portraits from the Old Testament.

James is a practical assignment to be carried out.

Peter is a course on physics, showing how the world may be blown apart.

John is the spiritual lapidary course for all students.

Jude gives a short course on the history of apostasy.

Revelation is a stereophonic preview of the world's last Saturday night.

Section 2
Articles About the Bible

The Bible

The **Bible** [according to the Christian arrangement*] contains 66 books written during the period of 60 generations. It contains the names of about 50 prophets, history extending over a period of nearly 4,200 years, and prophecy covering a larger period of 7,000 years. [*Note by author: The *Hebrew* Old Testament, the *T'nach*, has only 24 books.]

It speaks of about 23 different Nations and about 1400 Cities, Places and Countries (800 in the Holy Land); and it mentions nearly three dozen kinds of herbs, over a dozen musical instruments, 19 varieties of precious stone, about two dozen benighted heathen nations.

It also contains 150 songs of Zion, such as were sung by the Jews in their temple; about 100 kings and judges; about 30 high priests; about three dozen wars; and about 3,000 names.

–The Dawn

The Book

When Sir Walter Scott, who himself had written some three-score books, lay on his death bed, he asked his son-in-law Lockhart for "the book." "Which book, Sir Walter?" "There is only one book," he gave answer, and pointed to the Bible.

It is now some eighteen hundred years since there came into the world a book under auspices modest enough. No prospectus was sent forth months ahead to announce the forthcoming sensation; no posters were urging the passer-by to read the book, since every one else was reading it. It was not thrown into the lap of passengers in the railway coaches, nor were pictures of its author displayed in the shop windows. The Gladstones of those days wrote no lengthy reviews thereof. It was not dramatized for the stage, and was talked of neither at reception nor at club. So little stir did it make at its entrance into the world of letters that the popular dry goods seller of the day did not deem it worthy of being made a premium for every dollar of hose disposed of. Softly, silently it came; like all that is great, like every true gift from the heavens, like the falling snow, like the rays of the sun; yea, like the voice of Him that speaketh unto the heart of man neither in the thunder nor yet in the earthquake, but in the still small voice.

So softly indeed did this Book glide in that even unto this day, some eighteen centuries thereafter, no adequate name has yet been found therefor at the hands of men. As in its highest moments, the soul confesses before God that He is the Great Unspeakable, the Great Unnamable, so have men in their highest wisdom had to confess that this Book cannot be named, and it has ever since remained simply The Book, The Bible.

And yet this nameless Book somehow gets itself translated into every tongue, circulated in every clime; and read and studied, and lived by every age, every rank, and condition of life.[2]

The Textbook Says: ...... *But God Says:*

1. Man took thousands of years to discover fire.

1. God showed men fire: Tubalcain had a forge (Genesis 3:24, 4:22; Deuteronomy 5:24-25).

2. Man took thousands of years to discover metals.

2. Tubal-cain was a forger of brass and iron (Genesis 4:22).

3. There is no written record of how man got on earth.

3. God told Moses to write Genesis (Genesis 2:7).

4. It was a long time before man could talk.

4. Adam talked right away (Genesis 2:23).

5. Man's first home was in the forest.

5. God made the Garden of Eden for man's home (Genesis 2:10-15).

6. Man was afraid of the wild animals.

6. God brought animals to Adam (Genesis 2:19-20).

7. The first men had to hunt and kill to eat.

7. Everything Adam and Eve needed was in the garden (Genesis 2:9, 16).

8. Early men wore no clothing.

8. God clothed Adam and Eve (Genesis 3:21).

9. Animals had the advantage over man.

9. God gave man dominion over fish, birds and animals (Genesis 1:28).

---

[2]*The Writings of Ivan Panin,* p. 12, number 29.

10. Birth and death were great mysteries to men.	**10.** God taught men about birth and death (Genesis 4:1; Job 19:25).
11. Man came to believe in gods to explain life around him.	**11.** Man knew God personally–[he] came to believe in many gods because God gave him up to his foolishness (Genesis 3:8; Romans 1:18).
12. Man finally tamed some wild animals.	**12.** Abel tended flocks (Genesis 4:2).
13. It took man a long time to invent a boat.	**13.** God instructed Noah (Genesis 6:14).
14. The earth evolved over millions and millions of years.	**14.** God's seven-day creation [reconstruction] was thousands of years ago.

–Reprinted from *Brethren Missionary Herald*

Bibles With Strange Titles

by Reverend Earl Williamson[3]

In the past there have been a number of published Bibles bearing curious titles, some of which were:

Aching Bible: Oxford University Press once paid two guineas [42 shillings] for the loss of two letters in Matthew 26:55. The sentence should have read that Jesus was "teaching in the temple." By some strange occurrence the first two letters of individually set type were dropped out of the galley–the published copy read: "**aching** in the temple." Two readers made the discovery and claimed the reward for pointing out the error.

Bishops' Bible: This was the first "official" English version of the Bible, and was produced by a committee of bishops (1568 AD). It was an expensive edition, selling for about 16 pounds per copy. Being a poor translation, it never became popular. It practically fell out of use by 1606. Actually, this was the fourth revision of the Tyndale Version.

Breeches Bible, or **Geneva Bible (1560):** This was prepared by the Reformers in Geneva. It has Genesis 3:7 as, "They sewed fig

---

[3]*Biblical Research Monthly*, January 1975.

leaves together and made themselves **breeches**" (the London edition of the **Geneva Bible**, 1775, has "aprons"). This was the first Bible in which *italics* (for interpolations) were used, the first to omit the *Apocrypha*, and the first to be divided into **verses**.

Bug Bible (1549): Coverdale's translation of Psalm 91:5 reads, "Thou shalt not nede to be afrayed for **eny bugges** [or boogiemen] by night."

Discharge Bible: 1 Timothy 5:21 reads "I discharge thee before God," instead of "I charge thee."

Good Luck Bible (16th Century): Psalm 129:8, in Coverdale's Bible had "We wish you **good luck** in the name of the Lord." [From "The blessing of the Lord be upon you."]

Great Bible (1539): So-called because of its size; the pages were 9"x15". It was the first really Authorized Version of the Bible. By Royal Command of King Henry VIII a copy of the Great Bible was chained to a reading desk in front of every Parish Church in England; it was sometimes called the "Chained Bible," the "Cranmer Bible" (Thomas Cranmer, archbishop of Canterbury), the "Cromwell Bible" (Thomas Cromwell, Lord great Chamberlain), and the "Whitchurch Bible" (from the name of one of the printers).

Gutenberg Bible: Johann Gutenberg, of Mainz, Germany, is credited with inventing the printing press (1450). In 1454 he invented printing with movable type. The first book from the press was the **Latin Vulgate** (1455), called the **Mazarin Bible** because copies of it were found in the library of Cardinal Mazarin, at Paris. (A copy of the Gutenberg Bible is in the Huntington Library, San Marino, California. It is believed that there are 79 copies in existence, seven in the United States.)

He and She Bibles: Because in the **Vulgate** and **Syriac** versions Ruth 3:15 is rendered "**she** went into the city," some English translations read variantly "he" and "she." **Newberry's Bible** gives **he** in the text and **she** in the margin.

Leda Bible: Second edition of the **Bishops' Bible**, because of a woodcut used in it of "Leda and the Swan."

Mite Bible: The smallest Bible in the world. A reduced facsimile of the Oxford Bible, 936 pages, with illustrations. Only 1¾" x 1¼"; it is bound in real leather, with flaps and magnifier.

Murderer's Bible: So-called from a misprint of "murderers" for "murmurers" in Jude 16.

Palm Leaf Bible: In the library of the University of Gottingen (West Germany), written on 2,470 palm leaves.

Place-maker's Bible: Matthew 5:9, in the **Geneva Bible** (1562), reads, "Blessed are the **place-makers,**" instead of "peacemakers."

Printers' Bible: In one of the early printed Bibles this strange printer's mistake was made in Psalm 119:161: "**Printers** have persecuted me without a cause!" instead of "**Princes** have persecuted ..."

Standing Fishes Bible: In an 1806 edition instead of Ezekiel 47:10 reading "The fishers shall stand upon it [the river]," it reads: "the **fishes** will stand upon it."

Snowshoes Bible: In the translation for the Mumac Indians of Nova Scotia, Matthew 24:7 reads "A pair of **snowshoes** shall rise against a pair of **snowshoes,**" instead of "Nation shall rise against nation." The difference was made by one letter: "Naook**tu**kumiksijik," meaning nation; "Naook**ta**kumiksijik," meaning a pair of **snowshoes**.

Treacle Bible: So-called because of Jeremiah 8:22 being translated, "There is no **treacle** [an antidote against poison] in Gilead?" (Coverdale, 1535; Bishops', 1569). A few other curious expressions are: Genesis 8:11, "The dove bare an olive leafe in her **nebbe** [beak]"; Joshua 2:11, "Our heart had fayled us, neither is there good **stomacke** in any manne"; Judges 9:53, "And brake his **brainpanne** [cranium]"; Job 5:7, "Is it man that is born to misery like as a **byrd** for to flee?"; Acts 6:1, "Ther widowes were not looked vpon in the dyalie **handreaching**.

Vinegar Bible: An edition issued in 1717 had this headline to Luke 20: "The parable of the **Vinegar,**" instead of **Vineyard.**

Wicked Bible: Published in the days of King Charles I (1600-1649); it has the "**not**" left out of the 7th Commandment; a slip for which the English prelate, William Laud, inflicted a fine on the printers of 300 pounds. ["Thou shalt *not* commit adultery"–Exodus 20:14.]

References for above article:

Butterworth, Charles C. *The Literary Lineage of the King James Bible* (1340-1611). Philadelphia: University of Pennsylvania Press (1941).
Collett, Sydney. *All About the Bible*. London: Fleming H. Revell Co.
Encyclopaedia Britannica (1943), art. "Leda"–Vol. 13, p. 860. Chicago: Encyclopaedia Britannica, Inc.
Miller, H.S. *General Biblical Introduction* (1947). Houghton, N.Y., The Word-Bearer Press.
Pickering, Hy. *1000 Wonderful Things About the Bible*, London: Pickering & Inglis.
Webster's Biographical Dictionary (1970). Springfield, Mass.: G. & C. Meriam Co., Publishers.

The Bible is Full of Mistakes

by Winkie Pratney

The first mistake was when Eve doubted the Word of God;
the second mistake happened when her husband did too;
and mistake after mistake is being made
because people insist on doubting God's Word!
The Bible is full of contradictions—
it contradicts pride and prejudice;
it contradicts lust and lawlessness;
it contradicts your sin and mine.
The Bible is filled with failures—
because it is the record of people who
failed many times:
there was Adam;
there was Cain;
there was Moses;
there was David;
and many, many others.
But it is also a record of God's
never-failing love!

God did not write the Bible
for people who want to play
games with words;
for those who love to examine
good without doing it;
for the man who does not believe
because he does not want to.

Modern man has discarded the
teachings of the Bible
for the same reasons other men
have discarded it through history:
woeful ignorance as to its true
message and content;
determined apathy in refusing to
consider its claims;
parroted pseudo-scholarship posing
as honest criticism;
secret conviction that this Book
is right and men are wrong.

It is clear that only an ignoramus or
    prejudiced person would believe
    it teaches outmoded, irrational,
        unreasonable, and archaic principles;
        it is filled with hopeless discrepancies
        and unacceptable statements;
    it could only be the undirected,
        irrelevant, uninspired and
        unaided work of mere men.

The Bible is, after all, just another
    religious Book
    for thousands who do not dare be
        honest with themselves and God;
    for those who are afraid to accept
        God's own challenge to honest examination;
    for those unwilling to look in
        case it tells them what they
        are really like inside.

And you cannot understand or trust
    what the Bible says
    unless you are willing
        to consider the evidence
        and face up to the Author.

—*Accent on Action*

Great Books

The following very interesting information was carried in an issue of "California," State paper of the Mission Covenant Church:

A concerned housewife once wrote to a psychologist who had a regular column in the Chicago Daily News, saying,

"Some years ago I remember that Chancellor Hutchins of the University of Chicago stated that people are woefully ignorant of the great books of the past. He urged us to study them if we wished to become cultured people. So I've thought about organizing a 'Culture Club' for this purpose. Don't you think it would be a good idea?"

The reply from Dr. George W. Crane, the columnist, was as music to the ears of every true Christian who read it. He said:

"Yes, it is always desirable to improve your mind by good reading. Before you tackle Aristotle or Plato or other writers whom Dr. Hutchins glorifies, you had better read the four books that have had 10,000 times more influence on mankind than all these other volumes he advocates.

I refer to the four Gospels, Matthew, Mark, Luke and John, which are a small part of the Bible. The Bible contains 66 books under one cover. But most people, even with College diplomas, haven't read even the four Gospels in the New Testament! Yet those four books are responsible for most of the colleges in North America, and churches are simply living, functional Bible societies. Those four Gospels have also erected almost all of our hospitals, plus the Y.M.C.A.s and Y.W.C.A.s and C.Y.O. Halls.

Did you ever hear of a University created by Aristotle's writing? Or of a Plato Hospital? Of a William Shakespeare Youth Hall, or a Victor Hugo College, or a Goethe Salvation Army?

Facts No One Can Dodge

by *Keith L. Brooks*

Are you aware that there is one universally-translated and published Book having to do with the deepest heart-need of all people?

Its translatability into all languages and dialects in all climes and all ages–carrying in each one of them the same directness and authority, is the great puzzle of those who do not like this Book. *Man-made* books rarely bear translating into more than two or three languages, and even then lose their original force and fail to attract interest.

The BIBLE *alone* manifests its saving power wherever the Seed falls, in whatever age, for "it is the power of God unto salvation to *everyone* that believeth" (Romans 1:16).

Isn't it significant that this Book commands a profusion of readers over hundreds and hundreds of years that cannot be compared with the greatest works of the finest literary artists of history? No other Book in all history is so frequently quoted, so often printed. None has led to the writing of so many other books.

Were the 40 writers of the 66 sections of our Bible, who lived over a period of 1,600 years in widely separated areas–simply a succession of impostors trying to carry on a system of deception concerning God's redemptive purpose toward humanity? And has such a fraud proved to be the basis of the highest morality and purest spirituality known in history?

~ 12 ~

Miraculous Mathematics

Are you aware that these particular writings in the original Hebrew and Greek–the two languages in which each letter stands for a
numerical value–were so designed in their numeric structure that each
writer has left irrefutable proof that he was either an unparalleled
genius or must have been mysteriously guided by infinite wisdom?

Competent scholars who have spent years of research on the
numeric structure of these writings, have challenged the learned of
the world to produce one single article from human pen that can reveal
any numeric features comparable with those found in the Hebrew
and Greek of the Bible.

Are you aware that the very words, letters, phrases, books of the
Bible (66 books only) were so put together that they carry throughout
a most intricate numeric pattern, corresponding with those found
throughout all nature and the universe? These designs work out not
only on the precise count of letters and words, but on the totals of the
letter values. It is admitted that the writers, very ordinary men in
many cases, could not have *consciously* so written.

Will you deliberately deny yourself the available information on
such discoveries as this, simply because skeptical scholarship interested in promoting the theory of evolution, turns its back upon the
evidence?

Every Jew should know that every writer of his Old Testament
[*Tenakh*], regardless of educational background or circumstances, and
living without collaboration with the other writers–produced a marvel
in mathematics which, to modern mathematicians seems almost
unthinkable. How did they do it? And how did the writers of the New
Testament do precisely the same thing with the Greek letters?

The fact that this amazing numeric phenomena disappears if the
Old Testament is translated into Greek, or if the New Testament is
translated into Hebrew, is proof positive that the structure of these
writings alone came as the Bible itself asserts, when *"holy men of
God wrote as they were carried along by the Holy Ghost"* (2 Peter
1:21). Can any intelligent person afford to ignore such a Book?

Evidence of Archaeology

To what extent have you familiarized yourself with the amazing
discoveries of modern *Archaeology*? Are you aware that scores of
competent scholars in this field of science have turned up with their
spades in Bible lands untold treasures of evidence verifying practically
every part of the historic portions of the Bible? Have you ever read

any of the great volumes on archaeology that demolish the writings of skeptical authors and made ready for the bonfire, scores of books that have pictured Bible history as folklore and fairy-tale?

Every returning Jew in Israel today turns no shovel of earth to prepare the foundation of a home without looking for evidence, every piece of which is taken to the government Department of Antiquities. Here the most amazing proofs of Bible statements are being collected. One great scholar has said:

"The Bible waits at the head of the paths of scientific progress to greet the discoverer with its revelation of prior knowledge. The investigator climbs upward through the twilight and finds Scripture illuminating the summit of his climb."

Are you aware that *rationalism is a lost cause right now?* Do you know that, in the light of overwhelming evidence brought forth in the last 50 years, men who fume against the Bible and the Christian Faith are themselves the "Rip Van Winkles" who sleep as the evidence piles up?

Fulfilled Prophecy

Have you ever given consideration to the astounding evidence from fulfilled Bible prophecy, that the authors must have been directed by the only One who knows the end from the beginning?

No writings of men have ever contained prophecies comparable to those that make up almost one third of the Bible–prophecies reaching ages into the future and minutely foretelling the courses of ages. The Bible itself challenges all comers to consider its authenticity on the basis of fulfilled prophecy alone (Isaiah 46:9-10).

In our day the entire world scene fits in detail the prophecies as to how all men's schemes for building "one world" will reach their consummation. And what shall be said of the re-birth of the nation of Israel in the land from which she had been expelled for 2,000 years? The very line of division in the city of Jerusalem witnesses that the "times of the Gentiles" (Luke 24:21) are fast approaching their end. [This article written before 1948.]

Amazing Phenomena

Is it not obvious that God has given One Supreme Book to mankind? Can there ever be "One World" until human beings meet the terms laid down in this Book of books, through which alone men have found peace, hope, victory and all that makes for the highest well-being of man?

Fathomless Depths

If it is not HIS Book, how shall we account for its fathomlessness? No book of man has ever held the people of recognized intelligence age after age. No other book has ever stood up against the everchanging scientific theories of men and the philosophical speculations of the centuries.

Do you know anyone who has ever spent a long lifetime going into a minute study of any *human* literary production? Yet age after age some of the greatest thinkers give us the rich results of their research in the Bible, leaving thousands of volumes to witness to its infinite depths of truth.

Must it not be *infinite* wisdom between the covers of this Book that has withstood such concentrated hatred of men for 4,000 years, yet remaining like a Gibraltar to mock all the power of human genius, skeptical philosophy, atheistic ridicule and even the powers of heathen nations? If men produced it, men could destroy it.

Authoritative Standard

Have you ever stopped to think that we are living in a moral universe and that, just as certainly as a man reaps what he sows, and *more* than he sows, so in the life of the human being, man destroys himself and those about him if he does not conform to moral regulations that are suggested to him by his own reason and conscience?

Our great thinkers have long agreed that, if there is a moral order in the universe, then *somewhere* there should be *an authoritive standard* to which that order should be adjusted in order to function as it was intended by an intelligent Creator.

Where do we have such a standard, unless it is in the Bible, given by divine inspiration? If God has *not* furnished us such an authoritative source of instruction, He certainly *should* have done so, for it is not reasonable that He create individuals with aspirations that reach into the eternities, leaving them to grope in the dark for the way of righteousness and peace.

So perfectly has the Bible met this need in the lives of those who have submitted to its instruction, that there cannot be the slightest doubt but that this is the inspired Guide Book by which our course should be steered.

Witness of Experience

Only the willfully ignorant can have the hardihood to brush aside the universal voice of vital human experience that comes down to us through the centuries and is re-echoed by all today, of whatever church connection, who have met the basic terms of salvation, receiving the Lord Jesus Christ as their Sin-Bearer and Savior.

He was the One of whom the Old Testament prophets wrote centuries before His advent. He was the One who died upon the Cross of Calvary in fulfillment of some 159 prophecies. He was the One upon whom death could not get a grip and who arose and ascended to heaven to become the "One Mediator between God and man," the Final High Priest of God's flock.

Awaken a man to turn sincerely to the Gospel as presented in the New Testament - the realization of the same Gospel foretold in Isaiah, chapter 53, in the Old Testament and he will soon *find his own evidence* in the transforming experience of the New Birth (John 3:5,7) for "the Gospel is the power of God unto salvation to every one that believeth" (Romans 1:16).

"The preaching of the cross is to them that perish foolishness, but unto us who are saved, it is the power of God" (1 Corinthians 1:18). "If any man will do my will," said the Redeemer, "he shall know of the doctrine, whether it be of God, or whether I speak of myself" (John 7:17).

No Comparison Possible

So long as the Bible performs the necessary functions of a divine revelation and brings to those who whole-heartedly receive the Son of God as a personal Savior, "the peace of God that passeth all understanding"–can any fairminded person push it aside as of no interest to him?

Are you one of those persons who argues that Christianity is but ONE of the great religions of the world and that much good can be derived from other religious writings? Do you know of any of the so-called sacred writings of heathen religions that can produce any such evidences of divine inspiration as we have herein suggested?

What do these religions produce in moral and religious character? What have they done to raise the human race from degradation of *sin*?

On what ground can it be said that the literature of other religions deserve a place alongside the Word of God? Has Mohammedanism ever produced a man like the Apostle John? Has Brahmanism

[Hinduism] ever given us a Paul? Has Confucianism ever given us an Abraham or a Moses?

Find, if you can, in any of the heathen religions, or *in any of the false religious cults* professedly built on the Bible, characters like Luther, Wesley, Spurgeon, Moody, Carey, Taylor, Moffat, Livingston, or devout composers of sacred music such as the Christian Church has given the world!

Is it not apparent, friend, that the great reason the Bible towers above every Book and persists in spite of every device to destroy it or discredit it, is that it has proven productive of the highest type of human experience?

Key to Experience

Now, let it be understood that central in this marvelous volume is the Son of God, sent by the Father into the world to redeem all who "have sinned and come short of the glory of God" (Romans 3:23). His divine commission was attested by the prophecies of the Old Testament and by the miracles which He wrought, as well as by His resurrection from the grave.

He alone is the *key* to the experience of which we have been writing. The Gospel is very practical in its methods and the Son of God was always willing to have His claims inquired into. Obedience to His Word is the best commentary. Are YOU willing to put His salvation promises to the test?

"For WHOSOEVER shall call upon the name of the Lord shall be saved" (Romans 10:13).

"And they said, BELIEVE on the Lord Jesus Christ, and thou shalt be saved, and thy house" (Acts 16:31).

"That IF THOU shalt confess with thy mouth the Lord Jesus, and shalt believe in thine heart that God hath raised him from the dead, thou shalt be saved" (Romans 10:9).

Yes, it is as simple as that! "But these are written, that ye might believe that Jesus is the Christ, the Son of God; and that believing ye might have life through his name" (John 20:31).

Genuine Salvation

Whatever the alterations made by modern cults, sects and apostate churches—for, according to prophecy, these will multiply in the closing days of the present age—any one who *wills* may know what it means to be "born from above"—and, being "made a new creature in Christ," his own intuition will lead him to affiliate with some company of believers who *"earnestly contend for the faith which was once delivered unto the saints"* (Jude 3).

How Explain It?

After witnessing the victories of the cross for nearly two thousand years, how can it be doubted that *omniscience* was back of the Scriptures and that *omnipotence* is carrying them into execution despite all opposition?

We have seen that history and experience have both added an unimpeachable testimony. This Book of books has undeniably had a divine efficacy. Its words *are*, as our Lord said, "spirit and life" (John 6:63). They are "quick and powerful," (literally) "life-giving and energetic" (Hebrews 4:12).

Beyond the revelation of this Book, it is certain no human wisdom has ever reached. It furnishes the only truly rational and authoritative solution to all the perplexing and final problems of human destiny. The very contents of the Bible are such as to give an antecedent probability that *it could NOT be the work of the unaided human mind. It MUST be the Word of GOD.*

May the reader not forget that the primary purpose of this Book is to bring the assurance of eternal salvation to men–and that this is attained only through the atoning work of the Redeemer therein revealed. Are you robbing yourself of the wisdom that comes from above? Are you giving this Book the attention it deserves?[4]

"The greatest miracle of the Bible," says Dr. E. E. Slosson, a chemist of international fame, "is its chemical accuracy. The first book of the Bible says man was made out of the dust. In dust there are 14 different chemical elements, and in the body of man there are those same 14 chemical elements."

*NOTE: A more recent study reveals 16 elements but, no matter what study, if the same test is done on dust as on the human body, there are the same number of chemical elements in both.

The Bible Scientifically Accurate

In 1 Corinthians 15:39 the inspired writer tells us, *"All flesh is not the same flesh: but there is one kind of flesh of men, another flesh of beasts, another of fishes, and another of birds."* For a long time this truth was denied by biologists, who insisted that man's body descended from that of an animal. "But," says Dr. Rimmer, "there is now a biological reagent that will differentiate between tissues in the test-tube, classifying matter as animal or human. Regardless of whether the matter is living or dead, fresh or decomposed;

---

[4]Condensed from Keith L. Brooks' book entitled *The Divine Library:* "Proofs of Divine Inspiration."

bone or muscle, or any other section of what has been a vital creature; if this matter is placed in the receptacle, and the 'anti-human precipitin' is added, there is an instant reaction that states infallibly, 'This is human,' or 'This is animal.' Man can no longer be considered an animal any more than a canary bird can be called a fish!"

The Scriptures Divinely Inspired

by *John Wesley*

I beg leave to propose a short, clear and strong argument to prove the divine inspiration of the holy scriptures. The Bible must be the invention of good men or angels, bad men or devils, or of God.

1. It could not be the invention of men or angels, for they neither would nor could make a book and tell lies all the time they were writing it, saying, "Thus saith the Lord," when it was their own invention.

2. It could not be the invention of bad men or devils, for they could not make a book which commands all duty, and forbids all sins, and condemns their own souls to hell for all eternity.

3. Therefore, draw the conclusion that the Bible must have been given by Divine Inspiration.

Comparison

There is a unique harmony in the Bible. Take for instance a comparison of the first two and the last two chapters.
In *Genesis* the earth is created;
In *Revelation* it passes away.
In *Genesis* the sun and moon appear;
In *Revelation* there is no need of sun or moon.
In *Genesis* there is a garden, the home of man;
In *Revelation* there is a city, the home of nations.
In *Genesis* we are introduced to Satan;
In *Revelation* we see his doom.
In *Genesis* we hear the first sob and see the first tear;
In *Revelation* we read:
"God shall wipe away all tears from their eyes;
and there shall be no more death,
neither sorrow, nor crying."
In *Genesis* the curse is pronounced;
In *Revelation* we read: *"There shall be no more curse."*
In *Genesis* we see our first parents driven
from the Tree of Life;
In *Revelation* they are welcomed back.
—Author Unknown

Jesus and the Scriptures

𝕵 esus entered His earthly ministry with "It is written" and concluded it with the same note (Matthew 4:4, 7, 10; Luke 24:46). He accepted the OT Scriptures as the very Word of God. He stated that it must be fulfilled to the smallest Hebrew letter (jot/yod, ‏י‎) and to the smallest part of a letter (tittle) (Matthew 5:17-18).

In Mark 12:36, He used the phrase, "By the Holy Ghost," in relation to the OT, which is the regular formula used by the Jews of inspired literature. Never did He question the historical validity of the OT: Examples, story of Jonah and the account of Sodom and Gomorrah. Often did He refer to the fulfillment of OT prophecies, particularly those of Messianic importance (Luke 4:16-19 with Isaiah 61:1-2; Luke 4:21 and Matthew 21:4-5 with Isaiah 62:11 and Zechariah 9:9; see also Mark 14:21).

Messiah and the Old Testament

𝕸 essiah Himself bore testimony to the Old Testament in so many ways that it is impossible for any who acknowledge His authority to deny the authority of the Scriptures to which He appealed. He used them to defeat the Tempter, to confirm His words, to instruct His disciples, to correct the scribes and Pharisees; He insisted that the Scriptures must be fulfilled, and ascribed the writing of Psalm 110 to the inspiration of the Holy Spirit. On the cross He quoted from them and after His resurrection He expounded their teaching concerning Himself. Specially interesting is Matthew 5:17 and 18 where our Lord not only affirms that He did not come to abolish the law and the prophets, but to fulfill (plëroö, $\pi\lambda\eta\rho o\acute{\omega}$) them or give them their full meaning.

Oldest Book in Existence

𝕿 he Bible is the oldest book in existence; it has outlived the storms of thirty centuries. Men have endeavored by every means possible to banish it from the face of the earth: they have hidden it, burned it, made it a crime punishable with death to have it in possession, and the most bitter and relentless persecutions have been waged against those who had faith in it; but still the Book lives. Today, while many of its foes slumber in death, and hundreds of volumes written to discredit it and to overthrow its influence are long since forgotten, the Bible has found its way into every nation and language of earth, over two hundred different translations of it having been made (1974). The fact that this book has survived so many centuries, notwithstanding such unparalleled efforts to banish and destroy it, is at least strong circumstantial evidence that the great Being whom it claims as its Author, has also been its Preserver.

–Author Unknown

The Bible has 8,810 Promises

by Everek R. Storms

The Holy Scriptures contain a grand total of 8,810 promises. How do I know? I counted them.

All my life I have seen various figures quoted as to the number of promises in the Bible, the one most generally given being 30,000!

Since this is a round number with four zeros, I have always been a little suspicious about it. Furthermore, since there are only 31,101 verses in the Bible, it would mean that there would be practically one promise for every verse.

I do not guarantee my count to be perfect, but it is the most accurate I know of.

The Bible contains eight kinds of promises. There are 7,487 promises that God has given to man. This is about 85 percent of all the promises in the Bible.

There are almost 1,000 instances recorded, 991 to be exact, in which one person makes a promise to another person. This is some 11 percent of all the promises in the Scriptures. An example is the promise made by the Chaldeans to King Nebuchadnezzar: "Let the king tell his servants the dream, and we will show the interpretation of it" (Daniel 2:7).

There are also 290 promises made by man to God. The majority of these, 235 of them, are to be found in the Psalms, such as, "O Lord, open thou my lips; and my mouth shall show forth thy praise" (51:15).

There are 28 promises that were made by angels. Most of these (23 of them) are found in Luke. One example is the promise made by the angel to the women at Jesus' tomb: "Behold, he goeth before you into Galilee; there shall ye see him" (Matthew 28:7).

There are actually nine promises made by that old liar, the devil; e.g., "All these things will I give thee, if thou wilt fall down and worship me" (Matthew 4:9).

Two promises were made by an evil spirit. "Then there came out a spirit, and stood before the Lord, and said, I will entice him ..." (2 Chronicles 18:20-21).

There are also two promises made by God the Father to God the Son, and one made by a man to an angel.

One of the 66 books of the Bible has no promises at all–Titus (unless you count Titus 1:2 which antedates creation). Seventeen others contain less than 10 promises each. Even such an outstanding Book as Ephesians has only six promises.

The New Testament has 1,104 promises; the Old Testament 7,706. This means that seven out of every eight promises are to be found in the Old Testament. *You cannot afford to skip the Old Testament when you read your Bible.*

Isaiah, Jeremiah, and Ezekiel have over 1,000 promises each–a total of 3,086 in the three books, or more than one-third (35 percent) of all the promises in the Bible. Most of them are of a prophetic nature: "Behold, a [the] virgin shall conceive, and bear a son, and shall call his name Immanuel" (Isaiah 7:14).

Many verses have more than one promise. Here is a verse with four: "They that wait upon the Lord shall renew their strength; they shall mount up with wings as eagles; they shall run, and not be weary; and they shall walk, and not faint" (Isaiah 40:31).

Another verse has five promises: "Lift up your eyes to the heavens, and look upon the earth beneath: for the heavens shall vanish away like smoke, and the earth shall wax old like a garment, and they that dwell therein shall die in like manner: but my salvation shall be for ever, and my righteousness shall not be abolished" (Isaiah 51:6).

The chapter with the most promises is Deuteronomy 28. These 133 promises refer to the blessings and cursings God promised the Israelites when they would reach Canaan, according to whether they would obey or disobey His commands. A somewhat similar chapter is Leviticus 26, which has 94 promises, three-fourths of all the promises in the book.

The most outstanding chapter, as far as promises are concerned, is Psalm 37. Practically every verse in it is a most precious promise. Following are very few of these 43 wonderful promises:

"Delight thyself also in the LORD; and he shall give thee the desires of thine heart" (verse 4).

"Commit thy way unto the LORD; trust also in him; and he shall bring it to pass" (verse 5).

"But the meek shall inherit the earth; and shall delight themselves in the abundance of peace" (verse 11).

Last year I read the Bible through for the fifty-third time; but the time I read it counting the promises was one of the most precious. Time after time I have had to agree with Solomon: "... there hath not failed one word of all his good promise, ..." (1 Kings 8:56).

The question as to which are the greatest promises is one about which there would be difference of opinion. But if I were permitted to claim only six promises, I would choose the following:

The promise of salvation: "That if thou shalt confess with thy mouth the Lord Jesus, and shalt believe in thine heart that God hath raised him from the dead, thou shalt be saved" (Romans 10:9).

The promise of the Holy Spirit: "But ye shall receive power, after that the Holy Ghost is come upon you [the Holy Spirit coming upon you]: ... " (Acts 1:8).

The promise of answered prayer: "If ye abide in me, and my words abide in you, ye shall ask what ye will, and it shall be done unto you" (John 15:7).

The promise of temporal help: "But seek ye first the kingdom of God, and his righteousness; and all these things shall be added unto you" (Matthew 6:33).

The promise of sustaining strength: "... and as thy days, so shall thy strength be" (Deuteronomy 33:25).

The promise of heaven: "And if I go and prepare a place for you, I will come again, and receive you unto myself; that where I am, there ye may be also" (John 14:3).

If we had no other promises than these six, how good God would be to us!

The promises are ours for the asking–7,487 of them made by God himself. They are waiting for us to test and prove. We go to church and sing, "Standing on the promises," but most of us are simply sitting on them!

These are perilous times in which we are living. Recent developments in many lands emphasize this only too clearly. But the reply that [Adoniram] Judson gave his mission board when they inquired about the prospects for the future in Burma is still true for all of us: "The future is as bright as the promises of God."

You can count on the promises of God. Why not try some of them and see for yourself?[5]

---

[5]*Emphasis on Faith and Living*, Organ of the Missionary Church, Dr. Storms, editor.

Is That in the Bible?

by Christine Allison

*I*n the film *Beauty and the Beast,* a mob leader lays an ultimatum at Beauty's feet: "If you're not with us, you're against us."

Few will recognize this line as a quote from the Bible, a twist on Jesus' words in Matthew: "He that is not with me is against me." The phrase has been used countless times throughout history, even in the former Soviet Union by the likes of Lenin.

Biblical verse, especially as translated in the King James Version, has had a profound impact on our language, and variations of it turn up every day. Yet many of us quote the Bible *without realizing* it.

Even if you know the Bible, you may be surprised as you try to identify its phrases among these common expressions.

Old Testament

1. At a banquet, the Babylonian king Belshazzar saw:

    a) the light at the end of the tunnel.
    b) the handwriting on the wall.
    c) that the die was cast.
    d) that his days were numbered.

    Answer: b) Belshazzar, who showed no respect for the God of the Israelites, profaned the golden cups taken from the Temple at Jerusalem by ordering his companions to drink wine from them while toasting Babylonian idols. He was then amazed to see a disembodied hand, writing on the wall. The prophet Daniel interpreted the words to mean "Thou art weighed in the balances, and art found wanting" (Daniel 5:27). That night Belshazzar was slain.

2. Satan claimed that Job's virtue resulted from the material blessings God had granted him. To prove that Job's goodness derived from *his great faith*, God allowed Satan to test him by punishing him with horrible afflictions. Job's children were killed, his crops were ruined and his wealth was destroyed. Yet Job remained faithful, telling a friend that he:

    a) made it by the seat of his pants.
    b) escaped by the skin of his teeth.
    c) came within an inch of his life.
    d) would survive by hook or by crook.

Answer: b) Job actually said, "I am escaped with the skin of my teeth" (Job 19:20).

3. David, plucked out of obscurity to defeat Goliath and later to become king of Israel, begs God to protect him from persecutors. He asks the Lord to look upon him as:

    a) the apple of his eye.
    b) the jewel in his crown.
    c) his one and only.
    d) the fairest of all.

Answer: a) When David wrote, "Keep me as the apple of the eye, hide me under the shadow of thy wings" (Psalm 17:8), he was using a metaphor common in ancient times. The pupil of the eye, an extremely sensitive part and hence in need of protection, was thought to be shaped like an apple.

4. God chose Saul to be the first king of Israel. But when Saul began a forbidden attack on the Philistines, the prophet Samuel reproved him, saying the Lord sought:

    a) the last honest man.
    b) peace in our time.
    c) a man after his own heart.
    d) to put him through the paces.

Answer: c) And Samuel (1 Samuel 13:14) makes it plain this man "after his own heart" would not be the disobedient Saul but a newly chosen instrument of divine will. When God sends Samuel to find a new king, the prophet identifies David as God's choice.

5. Which adage is from the Book of Proverbs?

    a) A merry heart is as good as medicine.
    b) The rotten apple spoils its companions.
    c) Silence is golden.
    d) You can't cheat an honest man.

Answer: a) This bit of folk wisdom (Proverbs 17:22) has only recently been accepted in modern medical theory.

6. Moses grew up as a prince of Egypt and, after killing an Egyptian in defense of a fellow Hebrew, fled to the land of Midian, where he married and declared himself:

    a) rooted to the spot.
    b) a stranger in a strange land.
    c) at the end of his rope.
    d) out to pasture.

Answer: b) When his wife, Zipporah, bore him a son, Moses named him Gershom, which in Hebrew means "stranger there," for he said, "I have been a stranger in a strange land" (Exodus 2:22).

New Testament

7. Jesus began his ministry by performing miraculous cures that attracted huge crowds. Once when Jesus was surrounded by a multitude, his friends said he was:

a) out on a limb.
b) on the path to perdition.
c) beside himself.
d) on the side of the angels.

Answer: c) The press of the crowds and their response to his words affected Jesus deeply, for he seemed to go into a mystical state. "And when his friends heard of it, they went out to lay hold on him: for they said, He is beside himself" (Mark 3:21).

8. According to the parable, the complacent rich man reaped a great harvest, then said to himself:

a) Make hay while the sun shines.
b) That's icing on the cake.
c) Eat, drink and be merry.
d) A bird in the hand is worth two in the bush.

Answer: c) And God replied to him, "Thou fool, this night thy soul shall be required of thee" (Luke 12:20). This is what happens, Jesus explained, when a man grows rich for himself and not for God. The philosophy of "eat, drink and be merry" has its ups and downs in the Bible. Ecclesiastes (8:15) recommends it, "because a man hath no better thing under the sun." Isaiah (22:13) denounces it, adding the well-known appendage "for tomorrow we shall die."

9. Paul reminded his converts to resist the blandishments of the world, warning:

a) Beware the door with too many keys.
b) The love of money is the root of all evil.
c) Charity begins at home.
d) Where there's smoke, there's fire.

Answer: b) This may be the most misunderstood phrase in Scripture. In 1 Timothy 6:10, Paul does not say money is the root of all evil; it is *love* of money that destroys people.

10. One of Jesus' first public acts was to cast out unclean spirits. Challenged by a group of scribes who claimed that only with Satan's power could he cast out devils, Jesus rebuked them, saying:

    a) These words are sharper than a serpent's tooth.
    b) A house divided against itself cannot stand.
    c) This is the pot calling the kettle black.
    d) You will be hoisted by your own petard [case of explosives to break down a barrier].

Answer: b) "How can Satan cast out Satan?" Jesus asked. "If a house be divided against itself, that house cannot stand. And if Satan rise up against himself, and be divided, he cannot stand" (Mark 3:25-26). Abraham Lincoln made memorable use of the phrase before the Civil War.

11. Jesus once used this metaphor to make a point:

    a) Bend the tree while it is young.
    b) You can't judge a tree by its bark.
    c) You can tell a tree by its fruit.
    d) In a tempest beware the tree.

Answer: c) In Matthew 12:33, Jesus shows that one is judged by what he does, not what he says.

12. In one parable, a king prepares a lavish wedding feast for his son, but the guests don't show up. The king sends servants out to round up anyone they can find to attend. When one of the newly invited guests comes wearing inappropriate clothes, the king has him tossed out, saying:

    a) Do not play with fire.
    b) The clothes make the man.
    c) Many are called, but few are chosen.
    d) You add insult to injury.

Answer: c) In this parable, Jesus warned his listeners to prepare for the last judgment (Matthew 22:14). He was emphasizing a point he had made earlier: "So the last shall be first, and the first last: for many be called, but few chosen" (20:16).

13. After raising Lazarus from the dead, Jesus stayed with him and his sisters Mary and Martha. One night Mary washed Jesus' feet, causing Judas Iscariot to complain, and Jesus to answer:

    a) Charity begins at home.
    b) God helps those who help themselves.
    c) Cleanliness is next to godliness.
    d) The poor are with you always.

Answer: d) Mary had poured an expensive ointment on her Lord's feet, and Judas upbraided her for not using the money instead for the needy. Jesus said, "Let her alone: against the day of my burying hath she kept this. For the poor always ye have with you; but me ye have not always" (John 12:7-8).

14. When the early Christians were ostracized and attacked, the apostle James counseled them to endure these trials and show:

a) grace under pressure.
b) the patience of Job.
c) that one good turn deserves another.
d) a stiff upper lip.

Answer: b) James implored them to wait for the coming of the Lord, saying, "Ye have heard of the patience of Job" (James 5:11). Considering what Job went through, this could not have been a comforting allusion.

15. In the Sermon on the Mount, Jesus sought to inspire his followers with a new vision of their place in God's kingdom. He called them:

a) the best and the brightest.
b) babes in the woods.
c) the salt of the earth.
d) chips off the old block.

Answer: c) Key to preserving food, salt was one of the most valuable commodities in the ancient world. The phrase remains one of the highest compliments we can give another person.[6]

A Beautiful Tribute to the Bible

by Reverend William [Billy] A. Sunday, D.D.

Twenty-two years ago, with the Holy Spirit as my guide, I entered the wonderful temple of Christianity. I entered at the portico of **Genesis**, walked down through the Old Testament art galleries, where pictures of Noah, Abraham, Moses, Joseph, Isaac, Jacob and Daniel hung on the wall. I passed into the music room of **Psalms**, where the Spirit swept the keyboard of nature until it seemed that every reed and pipe in God's great organ responded to the tuneful harp of David, the sweet singer of Israel. I entered the chamber of **Ecclesiastes**, where the voice of the preacher was heard; and into the conservatory of Sharon, and the Lily of the Valley's sweet-scented

---

[6]*Reader's Digest*, July 1992, pp. 103-106.

spices filled and perfumed my life. I entered the business office of *Proverbs*, and then into the observatory room of the *Prophets*, where I saw telescopes of various sizes, pointed to far-off events, but all concentrated upon the Bright and Morning Star.

I entered the audience room of the King of kings, and caught a vision of His glory from the standpoint of *Matthew*, *Mark*, *Luke*, and *John*, passed into the *Acts* of the Apostles, where the Holy Spirit was doing His work in the formation of the infant church. Then into the correspondence room, where sat Paul, Peter, James and John, penning their *Epistles*. I stepped into the throne room of *Revelation*, where towered the glittering peaks, and got a vision of the King sitting upon the Throne in all His glory and I cried:

> "All hail the power of Jesus' name,
> Let angels prostrate fall,
> Bring forth the royal diadem
> And crown Him Lord of all !"

The Holy Bible for Girls and Boys

What a wonderful book is the Bible! It is the book of all books and the best book for boys and girls and all mankind. It is perhaps the oldest book in existence and the most circulated and best read book of all books.

The Bible has been translated into some 1,000 different languages and dialects and printed and circulated in practically every nation in the world. It is a universal book and the greatest traveler in the world. It is seen in the royal palace and in the humble cottage and read by emperors and beggars.

The Bible is God's Book; it is the Word of the Living God. The Holy Spirit of God is the author and every word is pure and true. "The words of the Lord are pure words; as silver tried in a furnace of earth, purified seven times" (Psalms 12:6). "For ever, O Lord, thy word is settled in heaven." "Thy word is true from the beginning" (Psalms 119:89, 160).

The Bible was written over a period of about sixteen-hundred years by some thirty-six men of God who lived at different times, in different places and were found in different walks of life. They did not write their own thoughts, or of their own wills, but as the Apostle Peter tells us, "holy men of God spake as they were *moved by the Holy Ghost*" (2 Peter 1:21). "Every scripture is divinely inspired" (2 Timothy 3:16, New Translation). Every word in the original manuscripts of the Bible, which were nearly all written in Hebrew or Greek, has come out of the mouth of the Lord (Deuteronomy 8:3), and was written down by men of God as the Holy Spirit moved them to write.

The Holy Scriptures are like a wonderful library of many books, sixty-six in all, and divided into two great parts, the Old Testament and the New Testament. In Luke 24:44 the Lord spoke of the Old Testament as containing the law of Moses, the prophets and the psalms, and that they all spoke of Himself. Thus we may say the Old Testament is divided into these three main divisions. ... Though the Bible is composed of so many different books of varied subjects, written by different books of varied subjects, written by so many different human instruments over so long a period of time, there is no contradiction in it. It is in itself a perfect book, though translations of the originals are sometimes faulty here and there. The Bible contains one harmonious story from beginning to end. The Lord Jesus Christ is its one great theme from first to last and the Spirit of God the one great Author that inspired every line.

Sometimes some people think that the Bible contradicts itself, but this is not true. The fault lies with the imperfect reader and not with the perfect book. Since God is its author, it is, and must be, perfect and without a mistake. But faith in God and the light of the Holy Spirit are needed to understand it; apart from this it cannot be understood.

All its sayings will come to pass, for the Lord Himself has said, "Heaven and earth shall pass away, but my words shall not pass away." He also said, "One jot or one tittle (the smallest of the Hebrew letters) shall in no wise pass from the law till all be fulfilled" (Matthew 24:35; 5:18).

The Bible is the only book that tells us all the truth about God, the eternity past and eternity to come. In it we learn about the past, the present and the future. It is the only book that tells us of the one and only, sure and certain way to heaven and everlasting blessing.

The Psalmist has truly said, "Thy word is a lamp unto my feet, and a light unto my path," and "The entrance of thy words giveth light; it giveth understanding to the simple" (Psalm 119:105, 130). It is the real map for the traveler and the true compass for the pilot.

The Word of God is compared to a mirror in James 1:22-25. When you look into the Word of God you see yourself and find out what you look like in the presence of a holy and righteous God. The Word of God tells us what evil lies in our hearts and that perfect looking glass shows us that we all are sinners and have come short of the glory of God.

But that same blessed Book also tells us of the remedy and payment for our sins. The Lord Jesus Christ is therein presented from beginning to end, in types and shadows and in reality, as the sinner's Savior who has shed His blood for our sins. Dear young reader, do you love the precious Bible and believe in the Lord Jesus Christ as your Savior?[7]

Bible Acrostic

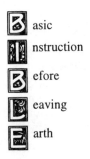

B asic

I nstruction

B efore

L eaving

E arth

Questions Answered by Ernest S. Williams

Some say that much of the Bible consists of fairy tales, and they point out that it mentions dragons and unicorns, for example–creatures that never existed. Are they correct?

Answer: They are not correct when they compare the Scriptures to fairy tales. The Bible does mention dragons and unicorns. In order to reconcile this with truth, it is necessary to understand that these are archaic words; that is, they meant certain things to readers three centuries ago when the Authorized Version of the Bible was published, but they have lost those meanings since that time.

May I quote from a paper published (eight years ago) by the American Bible Society:

> The **dragons** mentioned in the Bible are not the mythical oriental monsters we see in fantasy, but actually only jackals in Job and Psalms, though once the term may refer to sea monsters (Psalm 148:7).

> The legendary **unicorn** does not belong in the Bible for it is an archaic term for wild ox (Numbers 23:22).

---

[7] R.K.C. *Grace and Truth*, Danville, Illinois.

There are numerous other words which have changed in meaning or become obsolete. These are listed in the Appendix of the new English Reference Bible (King James Version) published by the American Bible Society.

For example, the KJV rendering "advertise" in Numbers 24:14 does not really mean "publicize," as one might expect, but "advise"; and "allege" in Acts 17:3 really means "prove." Few persons know that "bruit" in Jeremiah 10:22 is an old, unfamiliar word for which the modern equivalent is "report." When most of us see the word "charger," we think of knights and their steeds; actually, the word means the "platter" or "tray" which was used to carry John the Baptist's head to Herodias' daughter.

"Clouted" really means "patched" in Joshua 9:5 and "old cast clouts" means "worn out clothes" in Jeremiah 38:11,12. "Corn," used so often in the Bible, is well known to Britishers; but unless one stops to think about it, most Americans think of "corn on the cob" and not a general term for "grain" which is what is really meant in the Bible.

Who would guess that "emrods" really means "tumors" (1 Samuel 5:6); that "flowers" is a technical term for "impurity" (Leviticus 15:24); or that the "furniture" mentioned in Genesis 31:34 is really only a "saddle"?

Very often, the term "meat" in the Bible does not really mean animal flesh but actually "food" in general, even "meal" or "bread." "Outlandish" means "foreign" (Nehemiah 13:26) which one might guess if one stopped to think of the derivation of the word meaning "those from out of the land." "Polled" means "cut the hair of" (2 Samuel 14:26); "quick" does not mean "speedy" but "alive" (Leviticus 13:10; Hebrews 4:12). "Satyrs" are really "wild goats" (Isaiah 13:21), and "sincere" is "pure" (1 Peter 2:2). "Sod" is "boiled" (Genesis 25:29) and "tale" really conveys the idea of "talley" or "number" (Exodus 5:8).

"Skin of Your Teeth" is Real

SAN FRANCISCO, December 14, 1955–Dr. Louis J. Baume, assistant professor of dental medicine in the University of California College of Dentistry, has come up with some new findings about the "skin of your teeth."

The "skin," an enamel cuticle covering the enamel proper of the teeth, is found almost literally at the last minute before the tooth erupts, Baurne says.

The new finding not only throws new light on the formation of teeth, but it also may show how nature opens the way to a predisposition to tooth decay.

The "skin" is colorless, calcified, and about 10,000 of an inch thick. It constitutes the outermost defense wall of the tooth against infection, decay, and injury.

Scientists had believed that the cuticle is formed fairly early in the development of the teeth, long before they erupt. Baume found, however, that the cuticle does not develop until just before the tooth cuts the gum.

Baume studied the structures of teeth extracted from young monkeys before, during and after tooth eruption. He used a new tool, the phase contrast microscope, which enables him to see more detail of the structures than was possible with earlier techniques.

General Science of the Book of Job

Meteorology, including the aurora borealis (37:22-23), tornadoes (36:32; 37:1-5), dew (38:28), clouds and rains (26:27-29), snow, frost, hail and ice (38:22-23, 39), dawning of the morning (38:12-14).

Zoology: 1. Insects: The spider (8:14-15), the moth 4:18-19; 27:18). 2. Reptiles: The asp and viper (20:16). 3. Birds and Fowl: The vulture (28:7), raven (38:41), the stork and ostrich (39:13-18), eagle and hawk (39:20-26), owl (20:39). 4. Beasts: Camel, sheep, ox and she-ass (1:3; 42:12), lion (41:10-11), wild ass (6:5; 29:5-8), the dog (30:1), jackal (dragon) (30:29), mountain goat and hind (39:1-4), the horse (39:19-25), behemoth (hippopotamus) (40:15-24) and leviathan (or crocodile) (42).

Anatomy (34:15).

Geography, or the natural political divisions of the earth (Job 26:10; 38:18).

The Equator (38:5).

The Poles (38:6).

Mining Operations (28:1-4).

Natural Gas (28:5).

Writing, Engraving and Coining (19:23-24; 31:35-36; 42:11).

Scientific Facts Established

(Before Man's Discovery)

Isaiah 40:22–World a circle 3,000 years before man's discovery (1492).

Job 38:13–Four corners: East, West, North, South. Earth revolves around sun.

Genesis 2:21–Sleep in operation (chloroform).

Job 28:25–Weight of air.

Ecclesiastes 1:6-7–Wind circuit and clouds.

Job 26:7–An empty space in the north.

Job 38:35–Radio messages, electricity.

Genesis 15:5, Jeremiah 33:22–Stars unnumbered.

Job 37:7–Fingerprints.

Job 38:25–Path for electricity recently discovered.

Proverbs 24:3–Circulation of blood.

Job 25:5–Moon does not shine.

Genesis 2:7–Man, dust of the earth.

The Inspiration of the Scriptures Scientifically Demonstrated

Ivan Panin, a Jewish-Russian Christian immigrant, was a man of great wisdom and intellectual stamina. He loved the Lord and His Word so much as to undertake a long and tedious investigation into the Bible's authenticity as truly being inspired by God. He mathematically demonstrated that the pages could have been written by only One Author, even though having numerous writers. If the probable odds were calculated that what is described in Panin's document happened by "chance" alone, it would indeed be an astronomical figure.

At the turn of the 19th century, Ivan Panin wrote an editorial letter to the *New York Sun* in response to a challenge by a "rationalist" to present facts that would prove without doubt the Bible to be truly written by God Himself. In his response, he laid out specific numerical features within and correlations between the books of the Bible. For a group of men to have written the entire Old and New Testament books with these features would be a miraculous feat, if not impossible. Only God could have achieved so naturally this human impossibility. ... Mr. Panin demonstrated some numeric features within and between the different books of the Bible. The number *seven* is known as God's number, representing "completeness" or perfection. Mr. Panin found numerous patterns of *seven* throughout the Bible and presented these in two categories of "Facts": (1) numeric features within each book and (2) features between the books of the Old Testament. ... (There remains only to be added that by precisely the same kind of evidence the *Greek New* Testament is proved to be equally inspired.) Thus the very first verse of Genesis has patterns of *seven*–7 words, 28 letters, or 4 sevens; its very first syllable has a numeric value of 203, or 29 sevens–to name only three out of the dozens of numeric features this one verse of only *seven* words.

Is it possible that each writer of each book of the Bible was mentally capable of writing natural prose with such numeric precision and at the same time collaborate such that words unique to each of the books of the Bible have numeric patterns of *seven* as well? Unlikely. Impossible! But once one concludes that One Mind directed the whole process, the problem is solved simply enough–The Verbal inspiration breathed into the writing and canonizing of scripture is evidenced by this miraculously awesome feat. Every "jot and tittle" of the New and Old Testaments were authored by God Himself [through holy men whom He inspired].

Only in three ways can these numeric phenomena be refuted.

a. By showing that the numeric factors of *seven* as documented are not present in the words of the Bible.

b. By showing that it is possible for eight men to write each after the other seven; for 27 books [of the New Testament] with some 500 pages to be each in its turn written last (or they at least that they collaborated together in the scheme).

c. By showing that, even if the facts be true, the arithmetic fault-less, and the presentation of the numeric patterns honest, there is some other explanation besides the obvious: that men wrote them with inspiration from above. ...

As many as nine noted rationalists were respectfully but publicly invited to refute Ivan Panin. One was not "interested" in his "arith-metical" doings; two "regretted" that they "had not time" to give heed to it. Another "did not mean to be unkind," but ... . The rest were silent. For the special benefit of these, Mr. Panin printed the original data with numerous details, enabling them in the easiest manner to verify every statement made by him, if *they wished.* And to the best of his ability he has for years seen to it that no scholar whom surely these things specially concern remain in ignorance of the facts which he discovered.

I have a copy of *The Writings of Ivan Panin* which contains his scientific demonstration of the Scriptures in amazing detail. I regret that it is too lengthy to include here. But suffice it to say: he proved that the Bible was written in **sevens** and a multiple of **sevens**. Not only by the number of words, the consonants (some used as vowels) but because each Hebrew and Greek letter is considered also numerically, he shows that it could only be God who wrote the Scriptures through His anointed men of old.

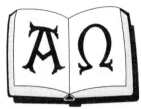

The Hairs of Your Head are Numbered

ome years ago a German scientist, with remarkable patience, counted the hairs on different heads. He took four heads of equal weight, and found the number of hairs according to Color as follows:

Red hair	90,000
Black hair	103,000
Brown hair	109,000
Blonde hair	140,000

Dark brown hair is by far the commonest in this country. It was found on investigation that out of a given number of people, 30 had red hair, 37 black hair, 108 fair hair, 338 light brown hair, and 807 dark brown hair. Surely such facts are interesting and can be used to profit. For instance, in a hairdresser's establishment one has read the apt notice: "Believe it or not, you have over 100,000 hairs in your head and we cut them all for a quarter." At this rate the baldheaded friend should have his few hairs trimmed at half price!

What wonderful things could be written about hair. Absalom used to cut his hair once a year, and the clippings, weighed 200 shekels after the weight, that is, 100 oz. avoirdupois. It would be a fine head of hair which *weighed five ounces,* but the mere clippings of Absalom's hair weighed 43,000 grains (more than 100 oz.). Strange, is it not, that the very thing upon which he prided himself brought about his tragic death!

When we want to express intense mental distress and astonishment we speak about our hair standing on end, a phrase borrowed from the Word of God. "The hair of my flesh stood up," Job 4:14-15.

Human hair has always been associated with strength, or with an outdoor occupation, as we read of Esau in Genesis, who was a "cunning hunter." And who has not been thrilled by the story of Samson, who lost his strength when he lost his hair!

Whether our hairs be white or black, brown or blonde, many or few, it is blessed to know that all the hairs upon our head are numbered. If tempted to doubt the minute care and provision of God, remember the fact that He has counted the strands of hair forming the natural covering of your head (see Matthew 10:30).[8]

Emotional Drunkards

It is a well-known fact that many movie-goers who are continually being excited and stirred in the world of "make-believe" become emotional drunkards.

There are also religious drunkards, Bible conference drunkards, and church drunkards, who go from meeting to meeting, constantly being stirred but doing nothing about it.

Their souls soon become "fed-up," their moral muscles deteriorate, and they lose their capacity for being aroused. Presently they suffer from a moral let-down, a religious hangover. They delude themselves.

They have heard the best preachers; they have read the best books; they have had their ears tickled and their emotions thrilled as with a stimulant; the doses have to be increased, so after a while there is no effect, no matter what they read or hear.

An alarm clock which fairly blasts us out of bed on the first morning may eventually fail to arouse us, if we continually ignore it. Something like that happens to those who join the band of travelers who hear–AND DO NOTHING !

–Vance Havner

When Paul was traveling on the Damascus road the Lord spoke to him from heaven:

*"It is hard for thee to kick against the **pricks**."*

The figure of speech is borrowed from a custom of Eastern countries: the oxdriver wields a long pole at the end of which is fixed a piece of sharpened iron, with which he urges the animal to go on or stand still or change its course; and if it is refractory it kicks against

---

[8]Dr. Herbert Lockyer in *Christian Reader's Digest.*

this goad, injuring and infuriating itself with the wounds it receives. This is a vivid picture of a man wounded and tortured by compunctions of conscience (fighting *against God*) which Paul was doing at that time.

* * * * *

(The following two articles were assignments for the class in *Poetical Books* at Seattle Bible College, Reverend Samuel T. Smith, Instructor. They were due and accepted on November 7, 1967. I enjoyed these studies very much.)

Proverbs

The word (Proverbs) in Hebrew is *mashal* meaning (in a good sense) either a maxim, a riddle, or a parable. The word is taken from the primitive root, "to rule," "to have dominion or power" (in intelligence or wisdom).

The title of this book is found in Proverbs 1:1-6 which expresses the purpose of these sayings–"to know wisdom and instruction ... the words of the wise, and their dark (or mysterious, hidden) sayings ..." The main content of the book is in praise of *wisdom*–the doctrines and instructions of the wise.

The very first mention of wisdom in Scripture is with reference to the Spirit of God (Exodus 28:3, 31:3). He is the true All-Wise One who possesses the power and dominion over all intelligences and wisdoms of the Universe. In the foregoing references we are told that when the Children of Israel were commanded to build the Sanctuary, they were not left helpless to obey. God gave them the spirit of wisdom that they might receive His instructions and be able to observe them. He also filled Bezaleel and Aholiab (the chief architects) with His Spirit that these leaders might, in the power of God's Wisdom, instruct the Israelites how to carry out every little detail in the way God desired it to be done. And this is the Wisdom which He has promised to each of His children: "Howbeit when he, the Spirit of truth, is come, he will guide you into all truth: ..." (John 16:13).

And how do we know that this is the promise of God? Through His Word. David said: "Through thy precepts I get *understanding*" (Psalm 110:104). He also said: "Thou [God] through thy commandments hast made me wiser than mine enemies," and "I have more *understanding* than all my teachers: for thy testimonies are my meditation. I *understand* more than the ancients, because I keep thy precepts" (Psalm 119:98-100). *Understanding God's will is KNOWLEDGE. Keeping or observing God's will is WISDOM.*

Therefore, to tell what wisdom is (in a good sense) and how to obtain it, might be given in these following few words:

Wisdom is knowing what to do and how to do it. This can only come by association with God, the All-Knowing and All-Wise One. We learn to know God's will and how to do His will by His Word through the Spirit. His Word is His will. The more we know His Word, the more we know His will and the more we observe His Word, His will, the more we obtain His wisdom!

The Song of Degrees

The Hebrew translation of "degrees" is "ascents" or "goings up" which would give it the complete title: "A Song For the Goings Up." This title would imply Jerusalem since the same term, "degrees," is used for "going up" to Jerusalem (as Jerusalem was on a moral elevation above all other Places). Literally, "A Song For 'The Ascendings"–viz., the stated annual journeys of successive pilgrims to the three great feasts in Jerusalem.

The Septuagint translates it as "Songs of the Steps." They are also called "Pilgrim Songs." G. Campbell Morgan considers these Psalms "as songs of which those pilgrims who went up to Jerusalem to worship, made use."

The Psalmist laments the conditions surrounding him as a sojourner and his soul is weary. He looks forward to the "land" where he can worship God and rest. The first two Psalms reveal the consciousness of the difficult circumstances of exile and the heart's confidence in Jehovah. The Pilgrim begins a long, toilsome march to the "city of God." The desire all the way through is to reach the dwelling place of Jehovah and to worship Him there. The last Song of Ascents (134) tells of rest which the Pilgrims have found for they have reached the Holy City at last, the activity of the day is over, and the priests in the Temple, who are performing their service there, are called upon to bless the Name of Jehovah.

The Jewish interpretation (contained in the Mishnah, the oral law which Jews believe was also given to Moses on Mount Sinai along with the written law) gives this description of the Temple:

"Fifteen steps led up from within it (the Court of the Women) to the Court of the Israelites (the Men), corresponding to the fifteen Songs of Ascents in the Psalms, and upon them the Levites used to sing (*Middoth* ii.5). At the ceremony of Rejoicing at the place of Water-drawing on the Festival of Tabernacles, the Levites were stationed 'upon the fifteen steps leading from the Court of the Israelites to the Court of Women, corresponding to the fifteen Songs of Ascents in the Psalms. It was upon these that the Levites stood with their musical instruments and sang their songs' (*Sukkah* v. 4). From these references the deduction used to be drawn that the 15 psalms received their title from these steps ... Since to go up is the verb used of the return from Babylon (Ezra vii.9), the suggestion has been made that the fifteen Psalms were composed for that happy event and sung by the home-comers as they approached Jerusalem."[9]

These fifteen Psalms were considered by G. Campbell as Pilgrim Songs and he gives the following titles to them:

Psalm 120–Jehovah, the Hope of the Pilgrim
Psalm 121–Jehovah, the Help of the Pilgrim
Psalm 122–Jehovah, the Glory of the Pilgrim
Psalm 123–Jehovah, the Helper of the Pilgrim
Psalm 124–Jehovah, the Deliverer of the Pilgrim
Psalm 125–Jehovah, the Protector of the Pilgrim
Psalm 126–Jehovah, the Restorer of the Pilgrim
Psalm 127–Jehovah, the Home-Maker of the Pilgrim
Psalm 128–Jehovah, the Home-Keeper of the Pilgrim
Psalm 129–Jehovah, the Confidence of the Pilgrim
Psalm 130–Jehovah, the Redeemer of the Pilgrim
Psalm 131–Jehovah, the Satisfaction of the Pilgrim
Psalm 132–Jehovah, the Assurance of the Pilgrim
Psalm 133–Jehovah, the Gatherer of the Pilgrim
Psalm 134–Jehovah, the Rest of the Pilgrim[10]

---

[9]*The Psalms*, Hebrew Text and English Translation with an Introduction and Commentary by *The Rev. Dr. A. Cohen.*
[10]From *Notes on the Psalms* by G. Campbell Morgan, pp. 248-264. The authors of "Songs of Ascents" is very uncertain. It is supposed that most of them were written by David, that Psalm 126 was written by Ezra, Psalm 127 and 132 by Solomon.

Section 3
Inspirational Truths

(The following *very brief* compositions are very *little* of what I have discovered in taking a "new look into the old book." Many other truths that the Lord has given me can be found in my other books, also is included elsewhere in this two-part book which I have written. I am continuing to find inspirational truths while I study God's Holy Word.)

In the Beginning

The very first verse in the Bible tells us that God was the Beginning. There is no question as to *how* He was, neither an argument as to *who* He was or *when* He was. Simply, His Word states *"in the beginning GOD."* He always was God and always will be God!

Our finite minds cannot comprehend what was *before* God in the beginning. We could ask some questions but cannot know or realize the answers. Was God all alone without earth, heaven, man, etc.? And, as a little child, we could ask "Who made God"? The answer would always be: "In the beginning God." There was not anyone before Him; neither was there anyone after Him. Simply, He was the "beginning."

God must have been "lonely,"–or could we say that this feeling was a part of Him? We will not know the reason He created man to be a companion in fellowship with Him until we reach Eternity. However, it has been explained by commentators and expositors of the Holy Bible that God created man to be His glory. For we do not say that God "needed" anything or anyone to accompany Him. However, the Scriptures do tell that God "brought into existence out of nothing that which would be glory for His Name."

*"Even every one that is called by my name: for I have **created him for my glory**, I have formed him; yea, I have made him"* (Isaiah 43:7).

We find the first verse in the book of John states what was in the beginning with God:

*"In the beginning was the Word, and the Word was with God, and the **Word was God.**"*

God was the Very Beginning and "*with* Him was the Word." This does not mean that there were two Gods, that God was not alone. This would seem to be a contradiction. But the Word was a *very part* of the **One** God just as you are *one* but one part of you is your spirit, one part is your soul and one part of you is your body. These are not *one* **and** one **and** one which would equal *three* but one **times** one, **times** one, **times** one is *ONE* !

> *"The same was in the beginning with God.* **All things were made** **by him***; and without him was not any thing made that was made"* (John 1:2-3).

The Word was the same with God and made everything that was made. Since God is one, yet three, it is God Himself, called the Word here, who is the Creator.

God Created the Alphabet

$\mathscr{J}$t is surprising to realize that before the heavens and the earth were created, before *anything* at all was made, God created the *Alphabet*! For how else does the *Word* appear? The Word is composed of letters of the Alphabet! Where do we read that God created the Alphabet in the beginning? It is found in the *Hebrew* text of the very first verse of the Scriptures as follows:

Be'reshith bara (תא) *Elohim*–"In the beginning God created תא (aleph-tav)," *i.e.*, the first and last letters of the Hebrew alphabet. When we abbreviate the *English* alphabet we use the first (A) and last letter (Z) to stand for the entire alphabet. There is no letter before A, no letter after Z. This is the same with the *Aleph-Tav*. It is the abbreviation of the entire *Hebrew* alphabet!

The Hebrew word for "beginning" is *reshith*. The ancient pictograph form for the letter *resh* (ר) was the back of a man's head. This signified the "head" or "beginning" of something. *God was the* **Resh,** *the Head, the Beginning.* The Word was **with** God and *is* God who created everything, even the Alphabet. Another way to say it is: *God created everything from A to Z.*

Where would we be without an Alphabet? For instance, we would not be able to communicate with others; and not being able to do this we could not build, travel, plan, invent, educate, etc. Just think of the many things which would be impossible to do without an alphabet!

Even God Himself *spoke* with the Alphabet He created to bring light to the heavens and the earth! The Jewish *Zohar* states:

"G-d looked into [the letters of] the Torah and created the universe. The Divine act of Creation is referred to by the metaphor of speech, as we say in the beginning of our morning prayers: 'Blessed be He who *said* ... and *the world came into being*." [Emphasis is mine.]

It was after God created the alphabet that the heavens and earth were brought into existence. Then God *said* (here His *Word* was spoken) "Light be" (Hebrew text of Genesis 1:4). He used the alphabet to create *light*. His Word, composed of the letters of the created Aleph-Tav, became **Light**.

"In the beginning was the Word, and the Word was with God, and the Word was God. And the Word was made flesh, and dwelt [tabernacled] *among us, ..."* (John 1:1, 14).

In the very beginning God created the Alphabet which He spoke to compose His Word. Then that Word which God spoke became Man as Messiah Jesus and lived among us "full of grace and truth, the only begotten of the Father" (John 1:14).

Not only was *Light* created by God's Word (composed of the Hebrew alphabet) but other parts of His creation came into actuality when God *said*, such as the following in Genesis 1:6-26:

And God SAID, Let there be a firmament in the midst of the waters, and let it divide the waters from the waters. And God SAID, Let the waters under the heaven be gathered together unto one place, and let the dry land appear: and it was so. And God SAID, Let the earth bring forth grass, the herb yielding seed, and the fruit tree yielding fruit after his kind, whose seed is in itself, upon the earth: and it was so. And God SAID, Let there be lights in the firmament of the heaven [sun, moon and stars] *to divide the day from the night; and let them be for signs, and for seasons, and for days, and years: And God SAID, Let the waters bring forth abundantly the moving creature* [fish, sea creatures] *that hath life, and fowl that may fly above the earth in the open firmament of heaven. And God SAID, Let the earth bring forth the living creature after his kind, cattle, and creeping things, and beast of the earth after his kind: and it was so. And God SAID, Let us make man in our image, after our likeness: and let them have dominion over the fish of the sea, and over the fowl of the air, and over the cattle, and over all the earth, and over every creeping thing that creepeth upon the earth.*

We see how God used the Alphabet which He created to also create the firmament, the waters, the land, the lesser lights (sun, moon, stars. He first created the great **Light**), sea creatures, fowl, animals, creeping things, and the last of His first creation: **man**.

A question is asked: "Why did God create man last and all these other things before him?" The Bible tells us that the creation of everything "from A to Z" was in preparation for the man who would "appropriate" all that God had made! As we study God's Word we find this outstanding fact: **the human being** is the highest creation of God. All else is made to accommodate this human's spirit, soul and body.

As we look into the Book to see new truths, we discover that the Alphabet which God created is a picture of Messiah Jesus.[11] From the very beginning of the Bible we see Him. God said (in the words made up of His created alphabet) that Light was to be. Who is the Light? In Messiah there is no darkness at all. He came to divide the darkness from the light. Jesus is the Light of the World who came to light every one who believes in Him.

*"Then spake Jesus again unto them, saying, **I am the light of the world**: he that followeth me shall not walk in **darkness**, but shall have the **light of life**"* (John 8:12).

Oh, I thank my wonderful Messiah who spoke His Word and shined His Light upon me! Thank God for the day God *said* to my soul "Let there be light" and the darkness in which I was walking was removed from my life!

When God looked upon His creation, especially the man He had formed out of the dust of the ground, He saw it was not good for him to be alone. Even as God Himself was not alone so He "considered" that the one He had created should not be by himself. Therefore, as man was to be made in God's own image and likeness, He made a "companion" for this man who would be his female counterpart. She was out of him to be like him and to be for him. This was a prophecy of the One who was to come. His bride, the church, would come out of Him, to be like Him and to be for Him.

God Reveals His Name to Moses

The first time God revealed His Name, not only to Moses but through Moses to all the children (sons) of Israel, is found in the following:

*"And Moses said unto God, Behold, when I come unto the children of Israel, and shall say unto them, The God of your fathers hath sent me unto you; and they shall say to me, What is his **name**? what shall I say unto them? And God said unto Moses, I AM THAT I AM [or **I will be what I will be**–Ayeh Asher Ayeh]: and he said, Thus shalt thou **say unto the children of Israel**, I AM [Ayeh, **I will be**] hath sent me unto you. And God said moreover unto Moses,*

---

[11]See my book, *Pictures of Messiah*, in the section: "Messiah in the Hebrew Alphabet," pp. 107-127.

*Thus shalt thou say unto the children of Israel, The **LORD God** [Yahweh-Elohim] of your fathers, the God of Abraham, the God of Isaac, and the God of Jacob, hath sent me unto you: this is **my name** for ever, and this is my memorial unto all generations"* (Exodus 3:13-15).

By the above Scripture portion we find that God did not withhold His Name from Moses, neither from the sons of Israel. He did not keep His Name a secret. The sons of Israel knew His Name and the pronunciation of that name as God revealed it to them. When Moses inquired as to God's Name, God unhesitatingly gave it to him! There is much that is involved in the Name of the Lord which we cannot enter into detail here. Suffice it to say that God's people (both Jew and Gentile) should know and pronounce His indescribable, glorious Name which involves many other Names of God even as Moses and Israel knew.

How thankful we should be that we can repeat God's wonderful Name (Names) and learn the meanings as it pertains to us in our life! God is not afar off from us in Messiah Jesus. All that is found in the Name of "Yahweh" is revealed to us by the Holy Spirit as we study His Word and walk in His way. As with Israel, the Name of the Lord is freely given to us to meet every situation and need in our lives.

My Jewish people today do not pronounce the personal eternal name of the Lord. The custom of writing this Name today is to leave out a letter so as not to use the full name: i.e., G-d, L-rd. They feel that by leaving out a letter they are not guilty of blasphemy or taking His Name in vain, as they interpret one of the commandments. It is to be regretted that this way of thinking is contrary to what their fore-fathers practiced.

In ancient times the Jewish scribes who were privileged to copy the Scriptures were very careful as they wrote the name of the Lord. When they would come to it in the Scriptures to copy it, first of all they took a bath, changed their clothes and used a new pen—it was that sacred to them. This procedure was followed according to the Talmud, not the Bible. When the scribes would do this they would go through the ceremony over sixty-eight hundred times—for that is the number of times the personal eternal Name of the Lord is found in the *Hebrew* text of the Scriptures! However, God never gave any prohibition for writing out His Name. If He did, we would not have the Holy Scriptures today with His personal eternal Name written out (in Hebrew) over sixty-eight hundred times! Also, when the Word of God was read in the Tabernacle, Temple and Synagogue, that glorious Name was *pronounced* without any prohibition! When the Messiah Yeshua came to earth He followed the Law of God and used the Holy Name when performing His miracles, or when He prayed to the Father or when He read it in the Synagogue! He taught His disciples to do the same.

God's Arithmetic Book

Addition: *"But seek ye first the kingdom of God, and his right-eousness; and all these things shall be **added** unto you"* (Matthew 6:33).

Subtraction: *"But now ye also **put off** all these; anger, wrath, malice, blasphemy, filthy communication out of your mouth. Lie not one to another, seeing that ye have **put off** the old man with his deeds;"* (Colossians 3:8-9).

Multiplication: *And every one that hath forsaken houses, or brethren, or sisters, or father, or mother, or wife, or children, or lands, for my name's sake, shall receive an **hundredfold** ..."* (Matthew 19:29).

Division: *"And before him shall be gathered all nations: and he shall separate them one from another, as a shepherd **divideth** his sheep from the goats:"* (Matthew 25:32).

Meek in the Bible does not mean "weak" as is defined in modern dictionaries. The Bible "meek" means "gentle," "humble," also "teachable."

Numbers 12:3–Moses was very meek.

Psalm 37:11–The meek shall inherit the earth.

Matthew 5:5–*Blessed* are the meek.

Matthew 11:29– (Jesus) "I am meek and *lowly* (humble) of heart" (see 21:5 also).

1 Peter 3:4–*ornament* of a meek and quiet (gentle) spirit.

The Dream

THE DREAM must *originate* with God, not man. (Abraham was called from Ur.)

THE DREAM will only work at the *proper time*. (Moses started 40 years too early!)

THE DREAM must be *dedicated* to the glory of God. (When God appeared to Moses the second time, the emphasis was on the "I AM," not on the servant.)

THE DREAM will always go through seeming *defeat* before the ultimate victory. (Joseph's prison and Moses' desert experience prove this fact.)

THE DREAM requires the driving force of *faith*. (Paul said, in the midst of the storm that threatened his dream, "It shall be even as it was told me.")

THE DREAM must not be *more important* to you than God. (God said that He, not our "Isaac," is to be our dream. All Isaacs in our lives must some day be sacrificed. God alone must be the source of our joy–our exceeding great reward!)
–Reprinted from *Life Share Pictorial*

Section 4
Answers to Some
Misunderstood Questions

From the cowardice that shrinks from new truth,
From the laziness that is content with half-truths,
From the arrogance that thinks it knows all truth,
O God of Truth, deliver us!
—*Ancient Prayer*

Cain's Wife–Where did He Get Her?

by Harold L. Proppe, B.D., M.A., Ph.D.

Cain's wife–where did he get her? This is an old question. It keeps coming up continually. Facetiously speaking, he got her where every married man gets his wife-from her parents.

Contrary to popular belief, the Bible is not silent on the subject but directly and indirectly tells us where Cain got his wife.

Before we study the verses in the Bible bearing on the subject we need to keep in mind some facts. One is that Cain and all his relatives lived in what we today call the Orient. In the Orient, persons marry very young or as in many instances, older men marry girls while they are still very young. Another thing to remember is that they did not then know anything of the practice of birth control as practiced by Occidentals. Married couples had large families. Reproduction was at a fast rate. The third thing to remember is that while the incidents and experiences in the Bible are Oriental in nature, the recording and preserving of those experiences and incidents are Jewish in viewpoint. In genealogy, the Jewish viewpoint is to record only the male members of the families, never the females. There were hardly any exceptions. Then too it is a custom and practice more so in the Orient than the Occident for cousins to marry. In some states in America first cousins are allowed to marry.

An Unlisted Number of Children

Keeping these facts and principles in mind let us look at some verses in Genesis.

Genesis 5:4: *"And the days of Adam after he had begotten Seth were eight hundred years: and* [-note this-] *he begat sons and daughters:"* Adam and Eve had other children besides Cain, Abel and Seth. There were *daughters.*

Genesis 4:1: In this reference we read, *"And Adam knew Eve his wife; and she conceived, and bare Cain, and said, I have gotten a man from the LORD."* It does not necessarily mean that Cain was the first child. The first child may have been a girl. In making a genealogy the Jewish people would begin with the male member of the family tree–hence Cain is mentioned, but no name appears of any daughters Adam and Eve had.

That the population of the world increased very rapidly in the Orient we know from Malthus' law.

A Sizable Population

That there were thousands of other persons, male and female, living at the time Cain went out, courted and married is clearly indicated in the following Scripture verses:

Genesis 4:14: "Behold, thou hast driven me out this day from the face of the earth; .. and it shall come to pass, that every one that findeth me shall slay me." .

Mark carefully these words: "It shall come to pass that *every one* that findeth me shall slay me." If Adam and Eve were the only other persons in the world then, Abel being dead, of whom then was Cain afraid? To whom does the phrase, "every one that findeth me" refer?

Genesis 4:15: And the LORD said unto him, Therefore whosoever slayeth Cain, vengeance shall be taken on him sevenfold. And the LORD set a mark upon Cain, lest any finding him should kill him."

Here God is speaking and we ask again, to whom do the words, "whosoever slayeth Cain" refer? Surely there were other persons present in the area where Cain lived to whom the "whosoever" applied. Again, to whom was God referring when he declared "lest any finding him should kill him"? Who was there present to find Cain and slay him? Why did God set a mark upon Cain? If there were no other persons living in the area at the time Cain was driven, by his own sins, away from God's altar, would not it have been simple just to tell Adam and Eve and warn them, without marking Cain?

The Holy Spirit, in superintending the recording of the events, saw to it that the right language was used to clearly indicate that the human race had multiplied itself to such an extent that an unknown number of persons lived in the vicinity to which Cain went to begin life anew. To whom else do such words as "everyone that findeth me"–"whosoever"–"lest any finding"–refer?

When the light of all the facts are gathered together and focused upon the old question, "Cain's wife–where did he get her?," the answer is: Cain had the opportunity, if he so desired, to court some 500 to 1,000 girls before he popped the question!

Someone was asked once what he did with those facts in the Bible which he could not understand? The reply: "I do the same as I do when I eat fish. I eat the meat and lay the bones to one side, and enjoy my meal."

Let us take David's attitude, *"Thy word is a lamp unto my feet, and a light unto my pathway."*

Train up a Child (A misunderstood statement in the Bible.)

"Train up a child in the way he should go: and when he is old, he will not depart from it" (Proverbs 22:6).

𝕵 understand *darku* not as a verb, "the way he should go," but as a simple possessive noun, "his way" (Proverbs 22:6). Simply put, **"Train a child in his [own] way; even when he is old he will not turn from it."** Let a child have his way and even when he is grown up, he will be a spoiled brat!

Too many Christian parents have mistakenly taken the traditional King James rendering as a promise of God and let their teen and adult children stray without a word, hoping in that promise of restoration. Parents should pray for and plead with their children who have turned away from faith. Proverbs 22:6 is a warning for child rearing.[12]

---

[12]Reverend Michael J. Imperiale, *First Presbyterian Church*, Greenlawn, N.Y.

Rapture or Destruction, Which?

Matthew 24:40-42

These verses are some of the ones most misunderstood in Scripture to many people because they interpret them in connection with the *rapture* instead of the *second advent*. It is quite clear from the context that the rapture is not referred to at all in Matthew, chapters 24 and 25. Therefore, regardless of how much these verses sound like the rapture of the church, they could not refer to that event. They refer to the *literal* [not the *secret*] coming of Christ to destroy the ungodly similar to the flood as is made clear by the use of the word "then."

> *"Then* [at the coming of Christ **with** the saints to end wickedness as did the flood] *shall two be in the field; the one shall be taken and the other left ... Watch therefore; for ye know not what hour your Lord doth come"* (Matthew 24:40, 42)

Why should we take these verses out of their proper setting which is at the coming of Christ *with* the saints, and make them refer to the coming of Christ *for* the saints? Why do we have to use this passage to prove that there will be a rapture or that some will be raptured from different parts of the Earth and some will be left? There are plenty of Scriptures to prove a rapture of some from the world besides this one ... Therefore, why should we base a doctrine upon a passage that does not concern the subject? If then, these verses refer to the *literal* coming of Christ, what do they mean? Where are these persons who will be taken? These questions are fully answered in the following passages which show that these verses refer to the *destruction* of some and the *preservation* of others at the *Battle of Armageddon*.

In Luke 17:34-37 we have a parallel passage to Matthew 24:40-42 which further proves that both refer to the coming of Christ *to* the *Earth*, and not to the rapture. The verses in Luke are the conclusion of a discourse concerning "the day when the Son of man is revealed" when two shall be here, and two there, the one shall be taken and the other left. This was a new teaching to the disciples, and they asked, "Where, Lord?" that is, they wanted to know where they were to be taken. The answer was, "Wheresoever the body is, thither will the eagles be gathered together." These statements in both Matthew and Luke are fulfilled at the coming of Christ *to the Earth*, and not at the rapture of the church. The Greek for *body* is *suma* meaning a corpse. The Greek for *carcass* is *ptoma* meaning a body fallen in death, a dead carcass [corpse]. Both Matthew and Luke use the same Greek word for eagles, *aetoi*, meaning the natural birds of the heavens (Revelation 4:7; 12:14). Thus if the passages were dealing with the rapture we would have Christ pictured as a dead carcass or corpse and saints pictured as living beings caught up to a dead carcass! This is beyond human conception, for neither Christ nor the saints are pictured in such a manner in the Bible.

Matthew 24:40-42 refers to the Battle of Armageddon when the angel will stand in the sun crying for the fowls to be gathered to eat the carcasses of men who have been slain by Christ and His armies at His coming, and who have previously been gathered to the battle, one from here and one from there (Revelation 19:17-21; Ezekiel 39:17-21). This picture of the eagles being gathered to eat the slain on the battlefield was a familiar one to the disciples. It is clearly described in Job 39:27-30. This mobilization of the hosts at Armageddon where they will meet death and make the supper for the fowls and beasts is pictured in Ezekiel 38 and 39; Joel 3; Zechariah 14; Revelation 16:13-16; 19:11-21. After this battle the carcasses of the hosts will lie all over the mountains of Palestine [now Israel] (Ezekiel 38:16; 39:2-5, 17:21), making a great feast as described in the above passages, *"For wheresoever the carcass is, there will the eagles be gathered together."*

This destruction is compared to the destruction at the time of the flood. Even as the flood came and "took them all away" ("destroyed them," Luke 17:27), so shall also the coming of the Son of man take some away and leave others to enter the Millennium (Zechariah 14:16-21; 2 Thessalonians 1:7-10; Jude 14).[13]

Added Notes to Preceding Article

In studying the Second Coming of Christ, it is important to distinguish between *The Rapture* and *The Revelation*, or the Lord coming *for* and coming *with* His saints. The one is a meeting in the "air" (2 Thessalonians 4:16-18), the other His coming to the "earth" (Zechariah 14:4-5). For the Rapture (Translation), see John 14:3; 1 Corinthians 15:51-52. For the Revelation, see Jude 14, Revelation 1:7, Matthew 25:31, Revelation 2:26-27. *Rapture*: Bride shown to the Father and angels in heaven. *Revelation*: Bride shown to the world.

"The Day of the Lord and the Day of Christ" cover the same time period (called "The Wrath of God"). "Day of Christ" pertains to the *people of God* during that time. "Day of the Lord" pertains to the *unsaved* during this same time period.

---

[13]Finis J. Dake, *God's Plan For Man, Part IV*, p. 24.

Can We Command God?

*"... concerning the work of my hands **command ye me**"* (Isaiah 45:11).

This is in the form of a question, not a statement of fact. Another translation which might be helpful is: "And would you question me about the future: Would you dictate to me about my work?" (Moffatt). It is presumptuous to think that man can force God to do that which is against His will.

But, moved by the Spirit of God, man might be emboldened to demand certain results. Do not forget that "we know not what we should pray for as we ought." It is only as one has the mind of the Spirit that intercession can be made *according to the will of God*, and that we may expect an answer (Romans 8:26-27).

Let us look at the context in the King James Version. First it says, "***Ask*** me of things to come concerning my sons, and concerning the work of my hands." Here we have God's advice to ascertain His will. Then He poses a question for the one who is asking concerning these things: "Command ye me?" Would you command Me about them?" No one can command or advise God about anything, least of all His plan for man, His universe, and future events!

Did God Give Israel Power to get Wealth?

Several years ago I listened to a sermon by a well-known evangelist intimating (during parts of his message) that Jews were rich because the Lord gave them the ability to acquire *money*. A Jewish person came with me to the service and was offended at what the evangelist suggested. In other words the evangelist inferred that this ability to acquire wealth was one of the reasons for anti-Semitism. I ask: why would God give the Jew the power to acquire that which would bring hatred to him?

To prove his point that God gave Israel power to get wealth, the evangelist quoted the Scripture verse:

> *"But thou shalt remember the LORD thy God: for it is he that **giveth thee power** [strength] **to get wealth**, that he may establish his covenant which he sware unto thy fathers, as it is this day"* (Deuteronomy 8:18).

We will examine the verses preceding this verse to understand the true meaning. The emphasis is on *work* not *faith*. Someone has said: "It is ***work*** that makes Deuteronomy 8:18 ***work***." By Israel's work with the *strength* [power] God gave them, they were able to bring the land into abundance. However, God gave them warning that they should not let this abundance from the good land make them proud and selfish. They were to feel their dependence on the Lord and not to think, "It is *my* power [strength] and the might of *mine* hand has gotten me [made for myself] this wealth" (verse 17). Verse 18 calls on the Israelites to remember that God gave them the strength (power) for work that makes wealth. And, true it is that most Jews (in nearly every field) work hard for what they earn. However, they are not to give themselves the praise but to *God be the glory*! This applies, not only to the Jew but to the Gentile as well!

Section 5
How to Study the Bible

Bible Study

There is *progression* in the Bible and it is good to follow a truth if you can, in your Bible, from the *beginning to the end*. There is always a place where that *truth* begins, and that is what Bible students call "the law of first mention." If you begin where God *first mentions* something and then trace that through the Bible you find how it expands until there is a place where God tells you *the whole story at once*. That is called the *"law of full treatment."* You have the love of God all through the Bible, but in 1 Corinthians 13 you have a whole chapter about God's love. You have faith beginning in Genesis 15, then a whole chapter about faith: Hebrews 11. Here you have "full treatment." It tells you just exactly what faith is.

There is progression in the Bible, and it is wonderful to follow it. In the book of John Jesus was alone *in the bosom of the Father* John 1:18. He came from the bosom of God. Jesus came to earth and He chose 12 disciples. Then, after He chose 12, He chose 70. Then in the book of Acts you have 120 in the Upper Room, and then later you have 3,000, and a few days after that you have 5,000, but in the book of Revelation, *"A multitude that no man can number."* You see, *it all started with the Son in the bosom of the Father.* When Christ left His place in the bosom of the Father it resulted in a multitude of sons that no man can number!

In Studying Your Bible Look for the Flags

Moody Press–Author Unknown

Some of the most important words of Scripture are little, daily used connectives that act like *flags* to call your attention to truths.

Recently I stopped at my bank to report I had mislaid my checkbook. The bookkeeper, clucking softly at my carelessness, told me she would "flag" my account. She attached a red marker to my account card and wrote on it, "SLost checkbook"–[See Lost checkbook] and the number of the misplaced checks. If a check came in against my account with the number of a missing check, it would be given extra careful scrutiny she assured me.

Likewise some of the most important words of Scripture are the little, familiar, daily-used "logical connectives" that relate to one another the thoughts or ideas of a passage. Whenever you see one of these words stop and think. The connectives are flags calling for your special attention. Ask yourself, "To what relationship does this word point?" To do so can open new vistas of Bible study for you.

This article is not easy reading. It is a study guide. Verses are not printed out. You will need to take your Bible and look up the verses referred to. The effort will be worthwhile if you develop the habit of scrutinizing the words of Scripture closely.

Connectives of reason explain why a statement is true. They occur either before or after the statement with which they deal. When you see one of these connectives, ask yourself what it is explaining.

BECAUSE: What statement in Romans 1:20 does the *because* in verse 21 explain? What three reasons follow the *because* to show why people are without excuse?

FOR (**because**): This short connective often has the same meaning as "because" and therefore deserves close study. It points to a reason for or an explanation of a statement that has been made. Note the series in Romans 1. What statement does the first *for* in verse 16 explain? You will gain better insight into these relationships of reason by putting into question form the statements that precede the *for,* using the word "why?"

FOR EXAMPLE: "*Why* was Paul ready to preach the Gospel at Rome?" (Because he was not ashamed of it?) "Why was he not ashamed?" (Because it is God's power unto salvation.) "Why is the Gospel God's power to salvation?" (Because in it God's righteousness is revealed from faith to faith.)

SINCE: This connective often has the meaning of "because," but it is used before, rather than after, the statement for which it gives the reason. It often means "seeing that." Notice 1 Corinthians 15:21. What reason (first part of verse) does this connective introduce for Christ's resurrection (second part of verse).

IF: Very often, but not always, this word is used with the meaning of "since." Look at Romans 6:8. Does the 'if' imply any condition, probability, or doubt? What main truth is being developed in the verse (second part)? What reason does the "since" introduce (first part) for believing this truth? Connectives of result indicate how one statement grows out of, rather than as a reason for, another.

SO (or *so then*): What truth is in view in Romans 9:16? In what way is it a result of something said in verse 15? What is the underlying truth in verse 15?

THEN: This word often means "accordingly" or "therefore." Look at Galatians 2:21 (in which the "if' does not mean "since" but implies doubt). Under what circumstances would Christ look at 1 Corinthians 9:12? What power, authority, or privilege had Paul and his associates not used? Why not?

Other connectives of contrast are *although* (Mark 14:29), *else* (otherwise) (1 Corinthians 14:16), and *yet* (1 Corinthians 5: 10).

Connectives of comparison show how two ideas or truths are similar rather than different.

ALSO: This word usually introduces an idea similar and additional to one that has been previously introduced. What basic truth is expressed in 2 Corinthians 1:21? What additional truth is introduced by "also" (vs. 22)? How is the new truth similar or like the one in verse 21? How does it go beyond it?

AS ... SO: This double connective compares two similar ideas or truths, the first of which usually illustrates the second. In Romans 12:4, 5, what truth (vs. 5) is being considered? How is verse 4 an illustration of this truth? (For other good illustrations of this usage, see Romans 5:18, 11:30, 31).

LIKEWISE (even so): Calls attention to a second truth as being similar to a statement already made. In Romans 6: 11 what truth is introduced by "how" is this truth similar to the one dealt with in verse 10? How does the previous verse throw additional light on the main truth? Other connectives of comparison include "also" (cf. Romans 9:25), *so likewise* (cf. 1 Corinthians 14:9), and *even as* (cf. Romans 4:6).

Series connectives join a number of facts, events or ideas together. Scripture begins with it. Often it has no special significance; you must decide whether or not it indicates a meaningful addition to a list as in Romans 4:11-12, 19 and 21.

FIRST OF ALL: This normally introduces the element named at the beginning of a series because it is in some way important. In 1 Timothy 2 what are the other elements in the series begun by this connective in verse 1?

LAST OF ALL: This phrase introduces the final element of a series—but sometimes the last position is reserved for the place of emphasis. In 1 Corinthians 15:8, for example, the connective could be classed as chronological but may also be considered as logical.

OR: This connective introduces an alternative, often with an element of comparison, as in 2 Corinthians 6:15, or of contrast.

The connective of condition introduces the stipulation on which a statement is based.

IF: You must decide, when you see an "if," whether the particle is used in the (sense) of "since," which is often the case, or to introduce a condition. Notice Romans 8:9a. Here the truth is that the believer is "in the Spirit." What condition or qualification does the "if" introduce?

Emphatic connectives are used to stress important points.

INDEED: Notice the use of this term in Romans 14:20.

ONLY (or *not only*): Examine Romans 4:9, 12; 5:3,11; 8:23, etc. for illustrations of how this term is used for emphasis.

Do you wonder, "Isn't all this bother about relationships a bit unnecessary? As we read, don't we automatically take in the meanings of the words and so, without any special attention to connectives, 'get the message'?"

To read the Bible is profitable, but to study Scripture, one must analyze, weigh, and scrutinize closely. To watch for connectives, to ferret [seek] out the relationships they indicate, to make the observations and interpretations and applications to which we have called attention in this series—this is to *study the Bible*. It involves time and effort—but the blessing always balances the effort and time spent in contact with the Word of God.

Section 6
Notes in My Bible

Soon after I received Jesus as my Messiah I inserted some notes in the Bible which my darling Mother gave me sixty years ago (1938). When this first Bible was used up with much of my collected material, I purchased another one and transferred these notes to it. Throughout the years: in Southern California College, during evangelistic services which the Lord opened for me to conduct, and the 23 years when I was an Instructor in Seattle Bible College, I continued to buy Bibles (since the old ones were worn out) to transfer the notes as well as adding some new ones. These notes are being reprinted in this present work to be transferred no more. My prayer is that you, the reader will benefit from this material and "take a new look into the old book." Following is the first item (by unknown author) I pasted in my Bible on the inside cover page:

The Bible

Never compare this Book with other books. Comparisons are dangerous. They speak from the earth, this speaks from Heaven. Never think or say that this Book contains the Word of God. It IS the Word of God. It is:

Supernatural in origin; Eternal in duration; Inexpressible in value; Infinite in scope; Divine in authorship; Regenerative in power; Infallible in authority; Universal in interest; Personal in application; Inspired in totality.

Read it through,
Write it down,
Pray it in,
Pass it on,
Feast on it.
Live it out.
It is the Word of God!

> *The Scriptures must be understood **grammatically** before they can be understood **theologically**.*

—Melanchthon

> While some books inform, and others reform, only the Bible can transform.

Be Ye Doers of the Word (James 1:22)

1) As the Engrafted Word it is to **be received** (James 1:21).
2) As the Faithful Word it is to **be held fast** (Titus 1:9).
3) As the Word of Life it is to **be held forth** (Philippians 2:16).
4) As the Word of Truth it is to **be rightly divided** (2 Timothy 2:1). *–Selected*

> Opening a Bible at random, putting a finger on a verse and allowing that verse to determine the course of action is called "bibliomancy," and is a form of Divination!

> The phrase: "Thus saith the Lord" appears more than 2,000 times in the Bible!

> There are from 5 to 10 thousand words in the *Hebrew* Bible.

> There are 1,189 chapters in the Bible. (These chapters were formed by the translators since the original languages of the Bible had no numbered chapters, sections, neither verses as we know them today.)

> The first book in the Old Testament (Genesis) ends with "a coffin in Egypt," the last book [Gentile arrangement] (Malachi) with "a curse." [The last book of the *Hebrew* Bible is: 1 & 2 Chronicles.]

> The first book in the New Testament (Matthew) ends with a promise, "Lo, I am with you alway" and the last book (Revelation) with the "grace of our Lord Jesus Christ be with you all."

Love for the Author of the Bible
is the best preparation for the study of the Bible.

Bible Study

The Bible deals with five great forms of study:

1. THEOLOGY, the science which treats of the existence, the nature and the attributes of God, and of His laws and governments, especially of man's relation to God.

2. ANTHROPOLOGY, the science of the origin and the nature of mankind, its division into various races, the classification, the relationship and the geographical distribution of the same.

3. SOTERIOLOGY, the science of the spiritual deliverance of the members of the human race from the guilt and the consequences of sin and death through the Saviorhood of Jesus Christ.

4. ECCLESIOLOGY, the science of the origin, the history, the purpose, the operation, the organization and the government of the Church.

5. ESCHATOLOGY, a theological term denoting the study of the last or final things, such as the Day of Judgment, the return of Christ to Earth, the Millennium, His setting up of conditions of eternity, and the state of the lost and saved when the present age ends.

—Unknown Author

The Best Thing To Do With the Bible

Stow it in the head, Sow it in the heart, Show it in your life,
For a STOWING, SOWING, SHOWING Christian
Is a GLOWING, GROWING Christian!

—Selected

Read the Bible

N ot as a newspaper, but as a home letter.

If a cluster of heavenly fruit hangs within reach, gather it.

If a promise lies upon the page as a blank cheque [check], cash it.

If a prayer is recorded, appropriate it, and launch it as a feathered arrow from the bow of your desire.

If an example of holiness gleams before you, ask God to do as much for you.

If a truth is revealed in all its intrinsic splendor, entreat that its brilliance may ever irradiate the hemisphere of your life like a star.

Entwine the climbing creepers of holy desire around the lattice-work of Scripture. So shall you come to say with the Psalmist, "O how I love Thy Law! It is my meditation all the day"!

—F.B. Meyer

T he Written Word tells of the Living Word Who makes the Illustrated Word. (The Christian is the illustrated Word.)

The Bible Remains

Many have butted their heads against the wall of God's truth and have thought it was tottering because they felt something give, but it was only their own heads that sprung. Many have gnashed on the Bible with their teeth and have thought they saw evidences that they were now gnawing the pillar down. The progress they have made is about like that of the rat that gnawed the file. He supposed he was making good progress because he saw the pile of white chips slowly increasing under his labor. But suddenly he saw blood and experienced pain, and then he realized that he had only used up his teeth. The Bible is a file on which many a rat has tried his teeth. They have gnawed for generations and made many chips. The Bible remains!

—Anonymous

Thought For Today

"No time, no time to study,
To meditate and pray,
And yet much time for doing
In a fleshly, worldly way
No time for things eternal,
But much for things of earth;
The things important set aside
For things of little worth.
Some things, 'tis true, are needful,
But first things must come first;
And what displaces God's own Word,
Of God it shall be cursed."

–M.E.H.

There was a time when they used to chain the BIBLE to the pulpit. Today I sometimes think it would be wise if they would chain the PREACHERS to the Bible.

—Reverend E. VanderJot

This Book will keep you from sin and sin will keep you from this Book.

—Dwight L. Moody

The Word of God

... has the power of the *sword*, sharp and piercing (Hebrews 4:12).

... is like a *hammer*, breaks the life so it can be pliable in the hands of God: (stony hearts broken in pieces).

... is like a *seed* (incorruptible), 1 Peter 1:23. Causes repentance, growth and change.

... is like a *mirror*. See image of God and ourselves (James 1:25). Shows us ourselves and the remedy to correct ourselves.

... is like *fire*–burn out those things unnecessary (Jeremiah 20:19).

The Bible Speaks

Just use me. I am the Bible. I am God's wonderful library. I am always, and above all, the truth. To the weary pilgrim I am a good strong staff. To the one who sits in gloom I am a glorious light. To those who stoop beneath heavy burdens, I am sweet rest. To him who has lost his way I am a safe guide. To those who have been hurt by sin I am a healing balm. To the discouraged I whisper glad messages of hope. To those who are distressed by the storms of life I am a safe anchor. To those who suffer in lonely solitude I am a cool, soft hand resting on a fevered brow. O child of man, to best defend me, just use me! —*Anonymous*

The Bible Stands

Century follows century–there it stands.
Empires rise and fall and are forgotten–there it stands.
Dynasty succeeds dynasty–there it stands.
Kings are crowned and uncrowned–there it stands.
Despised and torn to pieces–there it stands.
Atheists rail against it–there it stands.
Profane, prayerless punsters caricature it–there it stands.
Unbelief abandons it–there it stands.
Thunderbolts of wrath smite it–there it stands.
The flames are kindled about it–there it stands.
—*Selected*

The Word of God in the 119th Psalm

An Alphabetical Acrostic–A Messianic Symbol
Emphasizes the Word of God (John 1:1, 14).

All but six of the verses composing this Psalm make reference to the **Word of God** and in doing so, employ one or more of the following eight terms:

1. LAW. In the Bible this term refers quite uniformly to the "ten words" given by God at Sinai and the legislation growing out of them. [The term "Ten Commandments" is not found in the OT neither in the New. See Exodus 34:28 and Deuteronomy 4:13 in the **Hebrew** text where it is named "The Ten Words."]

2. COMMANDMENTS. Edicts Divinely given.

3. STATUTES. Details of Official practice founded upon the commandments of God.

4. JUDGMENTS. Decisions or court "findings." In the Scriptures, these three last named are frequently grouped together as comprising the whole Law, as in Deuteronomy 5:31 and 6:1.

5. WORD. This term as such, has varied significance, like some of our cognate English words. It is principally employed to designate the **Will of God** as expressed in the Scriptures.

6. PROMISE. A spoken word of assurance or response.

7. TESTIMONIES. Things to which God has borne testimony. Perhaps the word "intentions" would better express its significance. God's intentions are *in the nature of the case, prophetic.*

8. PRECEPTS. The root meaning is "to visit," hence "to charge," sometimes, "to punish." As used in this Psalm it seems to convey a more intimate and friendly meaning, as of fatherly counsel or correction.

—Author Unknown

The (119th) Psalm speaks about the *eternal* character of the WORD OF GOD. Three outstanding statements here contain the word *forever*.

v. 89. *"**For ever,** O LORD, thy word is **settled** in heaven [**present** truth*]."

v. 152. *"Concerning thy testimonies I have known of **old** that thou hast founded them **for ever** [looks into the **past**]."*

v. 160. *"Thy word is true from the beginning: and everyone of thy righteous **judgments** endureth **for ever** [looks into the **future**]."*

—Author Unknown

Verse Numbering in the Bible

Jewish Translations and the King James Version

There is a difference in some places of the Jewish translations from the verse numbering in the King James Version. Opinions vary regarding the first appearance of verse divisions, but the evidence seems to favor their introduction by the Masoretes. Robert Stevens is credited with following them in his edition of the Vulgate in AD 1545. However, there are some differences in the chapter and verse divisions which have been passed on down through the centuries.

These variations are too numerous to list here, but they are indicated in the margin of the American Standard Version of 1901 and in the New American Standard Bible. The first occurrence is in Exodus, chapters 7 and 8. Chapter 7 of the Jewish translations contains 29 verses so that chapter 8 begins with what is the fifth verse of chapter 8 in the King James Version.

As a result, chapter 8 of the Jewish translations possesses only 28 verses as compared with 32 in the KJV. In chapter 9 the numbering is again the same, and this continues until chapters 21 and 22 where another difference occurs.

The variations in some of the Psalms are due to the superscriptions. Some of these are considered as a verse in the Jewish translations so that verse 1 of the KJV becomes verse 2 in the Jewish. But this is not done consistently throughout. For example, the superscription of Psalm 139, "To the chief musician, a psalm of David," is considered as a part of verse 1 in the Jewish translations so the Psalm has the same number of verses as the KJV.

The same superscription in Psalm 140 is taken as a separate verse so this Psalm contains 14 verses instead of 13 as in the KJV. The superscriptions of Psalms 51, 52, 54, and 60 are divided into two verses in the Jewish translations so these psalms have two more verses than the King James.[14]

---

[14]Henry Heydt in "Questions and Answers," *The Chosen People*, American Board of Missions to the Jews.

Look At Me

Every time I look at me
I seem to see only me in me.
Please Lord, kick me out of me,
So that you'll find some room for You in me!

Humility is such a frail delicate thing that he who dares to think that he has it, proves by that single thought that he has it not.

–Ivan O. Miller

If I could crucify the flesh, that Christ in me might reign,
I must not spare my shrinking flesh the crucifixion pain;
'Tis either Christ or selfish I – what shall the answer be?
Let self be crucified that Christ, alone, might live in me!

—Max Reich

Cleanliness is next to godliness.
Carefulness leads to cleanliness;
Cleanliness to purity;
Purity to humility;
Humility to saintliness;
Saintliness to fear of sin;
Fear of sin to holiness;
And holiness to immortality.

–The Talmud

He who neglects *worship* neglects that which separates man from the birds, the animals, the insects, the fishes.
The unworshipful man is an anthropoid with a highly developed brain.
He may be a paragon of morality, but so are bees and ants.
Worship lifts men to the next level of experience and justifies their existence as men.
Intelligent worship is the most remarkable achievement of which a human being is capable.

—Dwight Bradley

Anyone can count the seeds in an apple —
but only God can count the apples in a seed!

God, the Eternal is thy refuge;
Let it still thy wild alarms;
Underneath thy deepest sorrow
Are the everlasting arms.
–Author unknown

It's not what goes in one's ear and
out the other that hurts,
but it's what goes in one's ear
and gets mixed up inside
and comes out the mouth!
–Lillian Rector

Freedom is the right to do that which the Law allows.

Divinely prescribed daily exercise for all growing children
of God:
1, 2, 3, 4,
Knees down, Body under, Faces up, Voices lifted!

No service in itself is small,
None great, tho' earth it fill:
But that is small, that seeks its own,
And great, that seeks God's will!
–Author unknown

If you cannot get all you want,
be thankful you don't get all you deserve!

When you have truly thanked God
For every blessing sent,
What little time will then remain
To murmur or lament !

It matters not the path on earth
my feet are made to trod;
it only matters how I live—
obedient to God !

The word "character" comes from a Greek word that means "to cut" or "to engrave." A character was a letter or sign that had been chiseled in stone or marble. Our character is the mark that has been made upon our personality by all our acts, habits and thoughts. Even as an engraving on stone remains legible for centuries, so is there something in man that will never perish, something engraved into his very being–it is his character.

People come in three classes:
>   The few who make things happen,
>   The many who watch things happen,
>   And the overwhelming majority
>   who have no idea what happened.
>   *–Selected*

His thoughts were slow,
>   And never formed to glisten,
>   But he was joy to all his friends–
>   You should have heard him *listen*!
>   *—Author unknown*

Perhaps that is why some of us do not get along better with other people–*we do not listen*. We are so busy thinking our own thoughts or listening to our own voice that we do not catch the message that others would like to communicate–by their actions, by their eyes, as well as by their words. People need to understand one another in order to have fellowship, and the way to get acquainted is *to listen* to each other. (Selected)

Nothing is quite so annoying as to have someone go right on talking when you're interrupting!

Remember, your tongue is in a wet place and is likely to SLIP!

Nobody raises his own reputation by lowering others!

DEAR ABBY: Believe it or not, I cannot find this information anywhere, so I am turning to you. *What are the seven deadly sins?*–Dumb Dora in Albany, N.Y.

DEAR DORA: Anger, avarice, envy, gluttony, pride, lust and sloth.

Seven Deadly Sins

*"These six things doth the LORD hate: yea, **seven** are an abomination unto him, A proud look, a lying tongue, and hands that shed innocent blood, An heart that deviseth wicked imaginations, feet that be swift in running to mischief, A false witness that speaketh lies, and he that soweth discord among brethren."* (Proverbs 6:16-19).

A brilliant re-classification of the old-time "Seven Deadly Sins" comes from the pen of **E. Stanley Jones**, who gives them the following titles:

Business without morality
Pleasure without conscience
Knowledge without character
Science without humanity
Politics without principle
Worship without sacrifice
Wealth without work

Growing Old

Lord, Thou knowest better than I know myself that I am *growing older*, and will some day be *old.*

Keep me from getting talkative, and particularly from the fatal habit of thinking I must say something on every subject and on every occasion.

Release me from craving to try to straighten out everybody's affairs.

Keep my mind free from the recital of endless details–give me wings to get to the point.

I ask for grace enough to listen to the tales of others' pains. Help me to endure them with patience. But seal my lips on my own aches and pains–they are increasing and my love of rehearsing them is becoming sweeter as the years go by.

Teach me the glorious lesson that occasionally it is possible that I may be mistaken.

Keep me reasonably sweet; I do not want to be a saint–some of them are so hard to live with–but a sour old woman is one of the crowning works of the devil.

Make me thoughtful, but not moody; helpful, but not bossy. With my vast store of wisdom, it seems a pity not to use it all–but Thou knowest, Lord, that I want a few friends at the end.

The above prayer was written by a Mother Superior who wishes to remain Anonymous.

—*Reader's Digest*

The People of the Book

The title "People of the Book" was first given to Jews by *Mohammed* but their interest in reading extends far beyond *The Book*. In Israel 2,000 books are published each year. Reading is really a national pastime. They keep 80 book publishers busy and bookstores seem to be on nearly every block in the larger cities. Besides all the books, Israel publishes daily 25 newspapers in many languages: Hebrew, Arabic, English, Yiddish, Polish, Bulgarian, Romanian, French, German, Russian, Hungarian.[15]

The Eight "Do More's"

1. Do more than exist, live.
2. Do more than touch, feel.
3. Do more than look, observe.
4. Do more than read, absorb.
5. Do more than hear, listen.
6. Do more than listen, understand.
7. Do more than think, ponder.
8. Do more than talk, say something!

—*Selected*

Importance of "Know-How"

A small midwestern city had trouble with its power plant. When no one could trace the difficulty, a hurried call was placed to Chicago and an expert soon arrived by plane. The gentleman examined the dynamo rather superficially, and then called for a small hammer. Slowly he started around the huge machine, tapping the hammer. Finally he asked them to start the motor again, and the machinery started whirring normally. The city officials were delighted until the bill for the trouble-shooting came from the expert. There was a charge of $800 for the very minor bit of work he did. Many thought it an outrage, and insisted that the man be required to give an itemized list of his charges. By return mail came a statement listing but two items:

Tapping the hammer 1.00
Knowing where to tap the hammer 799.00
Total $800.00

---

[15]*Jerusalem Post*, 1987.

> *Error* is truth out of balance!

> The *"Big-Bang Theory"* is: *In the beginning, a great Explosion!*

> *Sarah* is the only *woman* in the Bible whose age is given. She was 127 years old when she died (Genesis 23:1).

> *Rebekah* was Isaac's cousin. She was a Syrian [Gentile] (Genesis 25:20), sister of Laban (Genesis 28:2). (How could it be that she was a Gentile and her cousin Isaac was a Jew?)

> *Abraham* died when he was 175 years of age (Genesis 25:7).

> *Mount Zion* in Israel is a high hill outside Jerusalem walls, close by the Temple area but separated by a deep ravine.

> The word "remember" is repeated in the Old and New Testaments over *300 times!*

> *Og*, King of Bashan, (who was a giant) had a King-size bed! (Deuteronomy 3:11).

> Zedekiah's name before he ascended the throne was "Metanya" (2 Kings 24:17).

The Ten Commandments

TEN in *number* to express their divine perfection.
Written on tables of *stone* to signify their perpetuity.
They were written on *both* sides of the tablets,
as if to testify that *nothing* was to be added!

Teaching Jewish Children

The *Talmud* has laid the rule that when a child is *five years old* he must begin to read the Bible. At *ten* he must study the *Mishnah*. At *fifteen* he must study the *Gemarrah*. From that age on the higher study of rabbinical literature begins.

A *Yiddish* proverb states: "Wherever children are learning, there dwells the Divine Presence."

The *Talmud* says that Jerusalem was destroyed because the children did not attend school.

Jewish children brought up in an *orthodox* Jewish home are taught in the Bible, 6 hours a week. They are also taught all year long through their holidays and customs which are taken from the Bible account.

Doing Something Wonderful

When God is going to do something *Wonderful*,
    He begins with a *difficulty*.
If it is going to be something *very wonderful*,
    He begins with an *Impossibility*!

Plurality of "Elohim"

by Dr. Henry J. Heydt

Question: A Hebrew-Christian says that Deuteronomy 6:4 should be translated *"Hear O Israel, the Lord our Gods are one unity."* But I find in Mark 12:29, ASV, *"The Lord our God, the Lord is one."* I always understood that some Hebrew names for God were in the plural form and spoke of His fullness. Is that not right?

Answer: It is true that the Hebrew word for God in Deuteronomy. 6:4 is in the plural form, but whatever else may be its significance it certainly does not indicate a plurality of gods since the Hebrews were strict monotheists. For this reason our English translations never render it in the plural. The term poses a difficulty not only for the translators but for the expositors as well. Some have seen in it a remnant of polytheism, but God would never have used this name for Himself if this were its connotation. Others have thought that perhaps the plural is expressive of the fullness of the divine attributes, but this abstraction does not account for other factors such as plural verbs, pronouns, nouns and adjectives used with the name. These also militate against the Jewish explanation of "the plural of majesty." The *Soncino Chumash* has the following note on Genesis 1:1:

> "God. The Hebrew has the plural form, the plural of majesty; but no idea of plurality is to be read into the word, because the verb *created* is in the singular" (*Abraham Ibn Ezra*).

But this argument boomerangs because in Genesis 35:7 the *plural verb* is used with *Elohim*. Here Abraham Ibn Ezra finds himself in a noose of his own devising and attempts to extricate himself by saying that *Elohim* here means "angels," and this in spite of the statement, "and called the place ***El-bethel*** (the ***God*** of Bethel)!

The correct answer to the use of ***Elohim*** in Deuteronomy 6:4 with *'echad'* (compound oneness, a unity) is that within the one Godhead there exists a *plurality of persons*. This plurality is seen from other Scriptures to be three so that we have a tri-unity generally called a trinity.

Plurality and Unity

Hebrew	Translation
1. Baal	1. Master or Leader
2. Baalim	2. Masters or Leaders
3. Seraph	3. An angelic creature
4. Seraphim	4. Angelic creatures
5. Elohe	5. God
6. Elohim	6. Gods

"*Thou shalt have no other gods* [elohim] *before me*"(Exodus 20:3).
See Genesis 1:1 - "*In the beginning God* [Elohim] ..."

Hebrew	Translation
7. abhothenu	7. Our fathers
8. cholayenu	8. Our sicknesses
9. pesha'enu	9. Our transgressions
10. avothenu	10. Our sins

Elohenu — *Our Gods*

Looks

The *Psalmist* looks at your *hand*.
The *Phrenologist* looks at your *head*.
The *Doctor* looks at your *tongue*.
The *Detective* looks at your *eye*.
The LORD looketh on the heart.

What Became of the Children of Moses ?

Exodus 2:21-22

The Scripture indicates that they became absorbed into the Levitical service of the Tabernacle, since Moses, like Aaron, was of the tribe of Levi (1 Chronicles 23:14-15).

The Man, Moses

Moses is of all men the only one whom the Spirit hath condescended to liken unto the Lord Christ. A prophet *like unto me* shall the Lord declare unto the chosen people, and a right rich, a right full life he led, this man Moses.

Born in the house of toil, he is reared in a palace. Spends twoscore years at court, and fourscore in the wilderness. Leaves school without his God at forty, and is sent back to school by his God till he is eighty. Flees for his life, keeps sheep for a wife. Is alone forty years without a multitude, is alone another forty years with the multitude. Fasts forty days, and talks with God face to face. A rich life, a full life he leads, this man Moses.

A learned man, a wise man was this Moses. He was versed in all the wisdom of the Egyptians. The dynasties, he understood their puzzle. The hieroglyphics, he had fathomed their mystery. The pyramids, he had solved their problem. The sphinx, he had discovered its secret. A wise man, a learned man was this man Moses.

Come now, Moses, wilt thou not tell us what thou sawest those forty years at Pharao's [Pharaoh's] court? In the wilderness with Jethro, with Zippora thine, thy rebellious spouse, with Miriam, thy rebellious sister, with Israel thy rebellious people? Chevalier Bunsen would like to know. Professor Brugsch would like to know, plain Lepsius would like to know, the orientalists would like to know; scholars, historians, a host of cultured folk would like to know. Wilt thou not tell us, thou man Moses? But well nigh ravishing though these themes be, pyramidal silence is all he here hath for us, this man Moses. ...[16]

The Synagogue at Jerusalem was dedicated on August 4, 1982, in memory of the 6 million Jewish victims of the Holocaust. Claimed to be the most beautiful Jewish house of worship in the world, it is to be the central place of worship for Jewry worldwide until such time as the traditional site on the Temple Mount is restored.

Edom (Esau)–Mount Sier
Ezekiel 35:3-7

Petra, "The City of Mystery," has been called "The Rose-Red City as Old as Time," "The Rainbow City," and many other descriptive names suggested by its strange, desolate beauty. All we are able to find out about it from secular history is that it once had 267,000 inhabitants; that it was on a trade route from Egypt to Sheba, Iraq, and Persia; that it was inaccessible except through the RIFT (*Siq*) which was only wide enough for two horses abreast; and that the perpendicular walls of the Rift are from 400 to 700 feet high, and brilliant with all the colors of the rainbow. This beautiful city was occupied by the Nabataens from 100 BC until they were conquered by Rome about 106 AD.[17]

According to Daniel 9:24-27, the Messiah should have come apparently 2,000 years ago. According to Jewish writings:

---

[16]Ivan Panin, *The Writings of Ivan Panin*, pp.574-575.
[17]Joseph Hoffman Cohn, *I Have Loved Jacob*, p. 87.

"The *Tanna debe Eliyyahu* teaches: The world is to exist six thousand years. In the first two thousand there was desolation; two thousand years the Torah flourished; and the next two thousand years is the Messianic era, but through our many iniquities all these years have been lost." "He should have come at the beginning of the last two thousand years; the delay is due to our sins."[18]

Discover the Holy Place

by Floyd Wolfenbarger

When Moses met with God by the burning bush, he was commanded to take off his shoes for he was standing in a holy place. What was so sacred about the backside of a desert mountain? What made that particular spot "holy"?

Surely not because God was there, but because He is omnipresent, that is, He is everywhere. It could not have been because Moses himself was holy.

It seems to me that a holy place is *the place of encounter with God.* Wherever God and man truly meet is sacred.

Moses discovered that he needed no temple, no altar, no priest to be in a holy place. God visited him at work. Our home, shop, store or factory is holy if we *encounter the presence of God* there.

The Christian can discover the holy presence of God while driving down the highway in a pick-up truck. His prayers from his pick-up are heard by God as surely as prayers from a pew. He needs no organ music to lift his petitions toward heaven.

Moses was to remove his shoes because God had made him His servant in this holy place. The man who preaches the Word is often called the "man of God." However, the true Christian who sells insurance or lays bricks is no less a man of God. God has made the work of every Christian sacred. Whatever he does he must do for the glory of God.

Every labor of the Christian should therefore be diligent and honest. He cannot cheat his employer to the glory of God nor can a man oppress his workers without being accountable to the Lord.

For Isaiah it was the Holy Temple; for Moses it was mountain sheepfold; for Jeremiah it was a devastated city; for Ezekiel it was the refugee camp in the valley of Chebar. They learned that "the place

---

[18]*Sanhedrin* 97a-97b.

where thou standest is holy ground." Whether like Joseph we are prisoners or like Esther we rule, the work that we do is *holy work if done for His glory.*

A Word

WOE is a word of *Confession.*
    "LO" is a word of *Cleansing.*
    "GO" is a word of *Commission.*
                                    —*Selected*

Work without vision is mercenary.
    Vision without work is visionary,
    But vision plus work is *missionary.*
                                    –*Anonymous*

Isaiah 53 in Jewish Writings

In the *Zohar*, which is considered by pious Jews as the holiest of books, we read as follows:

"In the Garden of Eden there is one palace called 'The Palace of the Sufferers.' When the Messiah goes into this palace and calls to all the sufferers and grieving ones, all the agonies of Israel come upon Him. If the Messiah would not relieve Israel from the agonies and take them upon Himself, no one else could suffer the punishment of Israel for the transgression of Israel for the transgression of the law. As it is written in **Isaiah 53:4, 'Surely he hath borne our griefs'.**"

In *Siphre D'Bay Rav* we read:

"Thus saith Rabbi Jose of Galilee, 'Come and learn of the merits of the King Messiah who grieves for our transgressions, as it is written in **Isaiah 53:5: But he was wounded for our transgressions'.**"

We see from the foregoing passages that highly esteemed Hebrew scholars agree that *ISAIAH 53* plainly describes the Messiah who was bruised for the sins of the world!

The Key of David

We learn from Isaiah 22:22 in relation to the "Key of the House of David" that it was *placed upon the shoulder* as a sign of authority with the specific area being that of opening and shutting. This same significance is seen in the *Talmud.* We read in *Ta'anith* 2a,

"R. Johanan said: Three keys the Holy One, blessed be He, has retained in His own hand and not entrusted to the hand of any messenger, namely, the Key of Rain, the Key of Childbirth, and the Key of the Revival of the Dead. The Key of Rain, for it is written, *The Lord will open unto thee His good treasure, the heaven to give the rain of thy land in its season;* The Key of Childbirth, for it is written, *And God remembered Rachel ... and opened her womb*; The Key of the Revival of the Dead, for it is written, *And ye shall know that I am the Lord, when I have opened your graves.*" (So also *Sanhedrin* 113a.)

Points for Preachers

There is a great difference between a preacher and an *orator*. The orator gives what the books give to him, but the preacher gives what God and His Word reveals to him.

The real deepness in the exposition of the gospel is the fact of making it intelligible to all sincere hearts, even if they have no intellectual knowledge.

God is willing to do with any man or woman all that He ever did for any one. If there is not a mighty work of God in us, it is our own fault. Find out what the hindrances are and put them away.
–R. A. Torrey

Never rebuke a person until first you have wept over him.
–Ned Collingridge

God Did Not Call Me

(When I was called into the ministry shortly after I accepted the Lord [1938], I entered Bible College where one of my classes was "Homiletics" (the art of sermonizing or preaching). At that time, while being young in the Lord, I wrote the following composition concerning this. In later years I, myself, was given the opportunity to teach this same subject (Homiletics) at Seattle Bible College. But in my first introduction to the art of sermonizing as a subject I felt impressed to collect all that I had learned in the class and apply it to myself. As I read it over for this printing, I could see that this material seems to be judgmental and critical of the ministry. However, though it did relate to the unpleasant preaching and ministry of a few whom I had heard and met, my concern at that time was involving "my" own ministry. The title for the composition was: "I Am a Preacher But God Did Not Call Me." This was under my maiden name, Ruth Specter.)

God did not call me to tell funny stories to make the people laugh, nor to relate sad tales to make the people cry. My Lord did not call me to picture horrible incidents to bring fear to hearts. My good Shepherd did not call me to cut His sheep to pieces and beat them over their heads. The Mighty Counselor did not call me to give my own advise.

The Anointed One did not call me to criticize other preachers or denominations. The Great Forgiver did not call me to condemn or judge. He who was a Lamb "led to the slaughter, who openeth not His mouth," did not call me to defend myself or to argue. He who loves the unlovely did not call me to classify and choose those of His with whom I would associate.

He who washed His disciples feet did not call me to expect service from others. He who had no place to lay His head did not call me to a life of ease and comfort.

He who pressed Himself to pray alone–sometimes all night long–did not call me to wait for every convenience before I could afford any fellowship with Him. He who made Himself of no reputation did not call me to advertise myself. He who preached the *Gospel* did not call me to lecture on some great man, event, book, building, or invention.

He who came to seek and save the lost did not call me to sit at home and expect the "fish" to come to me. He who was anointed with the Holy Spirit did not call me to be an information bureau or an entertainer.

He who was "a man of sorrows" did not call me to be a comedian and a jokester. He, who through Paul, said: "Rejoice, and again I say, rejoice" did not call me to a sad countenance and a downward look.

He who is the Mighty Conqueror did not call me to be defeated. The King, whose child I am, did not call me to be a pauper. He who is the Resurrection and the Life did not call me to be powerless.

He who is our great High Priest and Intercessor did not call me to be unconcerned for those who do not know Christ. He who is our Master and Owner did not call me to live a life for myself. He who is the Truth did not call me to misrepresent Him in any way.

He who is the Righteousness of God did not call me to talk about my goodness. He who is the Worthy Lamb Sacrifice who shed His precious blood for the remission of my sins did not call me to accept or claim any praise or credit.

He who is the Miracle Worker did not call me to be "puffed up" when God performs a miracle under my hands. He who is the Holy

Temple of God did not call me to be light and frivolous in His "House of Prayer." He who is the great Deliverer did not call me to number the souls saved, healed, and baptized with the Holy Spirit in the ministry God has given me.

He who is called "Faithful and True" did not call me to count on crowds and offerings for success. He who is the Lord of glory did not call me to seek out leaders or moneyed men in order to "pull strings."

He who was meek and lowly of heart did not call me to exalt myself because of my office. He who took upon Himself a human form did not call me to take pride in my sex, race, or nationality. He who became a servant did not call me to consider myself better than others. He who chose a cruel cross, a thorny crown, and a bloody robe did not call me to a selfish life!

Hands for Jesus

Empty hands,
<blockquote>
Clean hands,
Quiet hands,
Anointed hands.
</blockquote>

> Christ needs your personality as a human channel through which to touch the men you touch.

> God speaks *to* men *through* men.

> So certainly as I must trust Jesus as my Savior so certainly must I constantly yield my life to the control of the Spirit of Jesus if I am to find real the practical power of His salvation.

> Messiah Jesus: The Word of God became flesh. The Son of God became man. The Lord of All became a servant. The Righteous One was made sin. The Eternal One tasted death. The Risen One now lives in men. The Seated One is coming again!

> In Jewish writings there is an interesting description of Laban:

"Laban is the perfect name for the person who functions as a mirror image to Jacob. When we write Laban's name backwards, we come up with *nun* [נ], *bet* [ב], *lamed* [ל], spelling *naval*, the Hebrew for *scoundrel*, Laban's true self."

However, in Scripture Jacob is not described by God as a scoundrel, but rather is pictured as a *perfect* man (*Ish Tam*), one who loved God, cherished his birthright, prevailed when he wrestled with God and whose name was included in God's very own name!

Endings of the Four Gospels

An interesting comparison of how the four Gospels end, each stressing a different aspect of Jesus' life and ministry was pointed out by Dr. Arthur Petrie, Bible teacher and writer. (Dr. Petrie was one of my teachers, also a fellow-teacher at Seattle Bible College.) This comparison is as follows: **Matthew** ends with the resurrection; **Mark**, with the Ascension; **Luke**, with the promise of the Holy Spirit; and **John**, with the Second Coming of the Lord.

The Law and the Gospel

The LAW commands
But gives me neither feet nor hands -
A better thing The GOSPEL brings,
It bids me fly And gives me wings!
—Selected

Views of Christ

Mark gives a general view of the Christ;
Matthew, the Jewish;
that by **St. Luke**, the Gentile;
and that by **St. John**, the Church's view.

> The New Testament has an overwhelming number of Greek copies and early versions which number about 24,633!

> Hagar named God אל ראי (*El Roi*), "A God of Seeing" (Genesis 16:13).

Prayers

God looks not at the *oratory* of your prayers, how elegant they may be; nor at the *geometry* of your prayers, how long they may be; nor at the *arithmetic* of your prayers, how many they may be; nor at the *logic* of your prayers, how methodical they may be; but He looks at their *sincerity*. *–Selected*

> *Prayer* is not a monologue, but a dialogue; God's voice in response to mine is its most important part!

> In His humanity Jesus had brothers and sisters. *"Is not this the carpenter's son? Is not his mother called Mary? and his **brethren**, James, and Josea, and Simon, and Judas? And his **sisters**, are they not all with us? ..."* (Matthew 13:55-56. Also Galatians 1:19).

Redemption

𝕿he Father planned it (Ephesians 1:4).
The Son purchased it (Ephesians 1:7).
The Holy Spirit processed it (Ephesians 1:12).

Scarlet Thread

𝕿*amar* was the mother of twins; one who came out first was marked (by the midwife) with a scarlet thread around his hand.

"And it came to pass, when she travailed, that the one put out his hand: and the midwife took and bound upon his hand a scarlet thread, saying, This came out first" (Genesis 38:28).

> All the curses that King David spoke against Joab eventually found fulfillment among David's descendants.[19]

Study to be Quiet

*"And that ye **study to be quiet**, and to do your own business, and to work with your own hands, as we commanded you;* (1Thessalonians 4:11).

𝕾tudy to be quiet–that inner tranquility that does not cause disturbance in other people–that honor bestowed by God on the inner man that does not show off so that others are disturbed or upset.

𝖂hen the crucifixion of Messiah was completed ("It is finished," "fulfilled," "done"), the law of Moses and the Old Covenant was fulfilled and satisfied (Hebrews 8:1-13; 10:1-22) and a New Covenant established (Matthew 26:28; Hebrews 8:7-13). We see in this that the New Covenant replaces the (Old) First Covenant.

God would make this New Covenant with Israel (Jeremiah 31:31-34) and this Covenant (not Law) would be expanded to include the Gentiles (Isaiah 60:3)!

---

[19]Talmud, *Sanhedrin* 48b.

Vinegar and Water

Why was Christ offered vinegar and water when he was dying on the cross?

The Roman soldiers were offering Christ the "canteen" of the Roman army–a sponge soaked in vinegar and water. Each soldier was issued a sponge which he soaked with vinegar and water and placed inside his helmet. This helped the soldiers overcome the heat and provided a cushion against blows on the head. The combination of vinegar and water was the soldier's normal field drink and was known as "posea." In addition to adding flavor to the water, the vinegar was considered to be a purifier.[20]

> The story of Passover celebrated in Jewish communities is read from "The Haggadah" which was written around 300 AD and today has over 3,500 editions.

Lapidary is the title applied to a workman in the art of cutting, polishing and engraving precious stones.

"It is curious to observe, in connection with the *almond*-bowl of the golden lampstand, that in the language of *lapidaries*, are pieces of rock-crystal even now used in adorning branch candlesticks (and hanging chandeliers)."[21]

The Midwest of the United States of America is called the "Bible Belt" because five evangelical denominations are headquartered in Illinois, five more in Indiana, and eight in Missouri.

The Other Three R's

Reason, **R**esearch, and **R**evelation. These can be reduced to *philosophy*, *science* and *religion*. In elementary schools we somewhat master the three R's, but the *other* three R's we grapple with throughout life.

—Author unknown

Born Again

Many neglect the born-again experience because they can't understand it. But a baby doesn't have to understand embryology to be born. You don't have to understand theology to be born again, any more than you have to understand botany to appreciate a tulip or entomology to gaze with wonder at a butterfly.

—Selected

---

[20]Reprinted from *The Los Angeles Herald and Examiner*.
[21]*Smith's Bible Dictionary*.

Pray for Peace

(God is pro-Israel in the sense that He is Anti-Arab ... No national power will overcome her [Israel], not because of her great military accomplishments or her high moral standards of her genius, but because God has a role for her to play ... Islam is strong because Christianity is so weak ... If Christians would begin to use the power that is theirs through prayer then the grip that Satan has on the 130 million Arabs would be broken ... *Do not bother praying for the peace of Jerusalem unless you are willing to pray for the peace of Damascus, Amman, Riyadh or Cairo* ... Today in the Arab world there is less than one evangelical missionary for every 10 million people ... The Jew and the Arab will be at peace with each other *only* when the Prince of Peace is in His rightful place in our hearts as well as theirs ...[22]

Peace in the Middle East ?

*"In that day shall there be a highway out of Egypt to Assyria, and the Assyrian shall come into Egypt, and the Egyptian into Assyria, and the Egyptians shall serve with the Assyrians. In that day shall Israel be the third with Egypt and with Assyria, even a blessing in the midst of the land: Whom the LORD of hosts shall bless, saying, **Blessed be Egypt my people, and Assyria the work of my hands, and Israel mine inheritance"** (Isaiah 19:23-25).*

Milk and Honey

(The reference in the Bible is not to **bee honey** but to **date honey**. The Jews include the date among the seven agricultural species which are "the glory of the land of Israel" (Deuteronomy 8:8). The seven species includes *d'vash* or honey, meaning date honey, gives the "date" a place among the seven species. Exodus 13:5–*d'vash*, "the honey of figs or dates."

The Mishnah (Oral Law) states that the "milk" is not milk and the honey is not honey. The Mishnah declares that "a land flowing with milk and honey" means "that the fruits should be tasty." The phrase applies to the *quality* of the fruits of Israel.

---

[22]Excerpts from a letter by Doug Sparks, Middle East Director of *Youth With a Mission.*

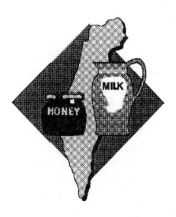

Joel 4:18–"The hills shall flow with milk"–not literal milk. Song of Songs 4:11–"Honey and milk are under thy tongue." Does not mean that she has taken a sip of milk and not yet swallowed it; nor that she has literally provided herself with a "honeyed tongue"! It is beyond question a metaphor for the fragrance of her kisses. If, therefore, "milk and honey" is found in this passage as a metaphor for *fragrance* and *sweet taste*, the rabbis probably were right in interpreting the oft-repeated phrase, *"A land flowing with milk and honey"* as meaning *"A land whose fruits are tasty and fragrant."* Israel is a land which produces not only fruit in *abundance*, but *delicious* fruit.

Part 2

Be in Health

This part is dedicated to my
Yahweh-Rapha — The Lord who heals

The following items which pertain to healing for spirit, soul and body I have collected throughout the years since I accepted Yeshua as my Messiah (1938). Most of this material is taken from the Scriptures to be applied to God's people. To the best of the ability given to me by the Lord, I have put to use the helpful and wise advice in some of these writings. I realize that the Lord is my great Physician, my *Yahweh Rapha* and I have benefited by using His Medicine Chest (the Bible) for all my spiritual, physical, mental and material needs. My age is 82 at this writing and I am in excellent health. Praise be to the Lord for this gift of His love!

The Yiddish term similar to "be in health" is *tzu gezunt* and when we were children we would hear it especially after we had sneezed! It is likened to a prayer for the individual to be healthy. My prayers for you, the reader, are found in God's Word:

"Beloved, I wish above all things that thou mayest prosper and be in health, even as thy soul prospereth" (3 John 1:2).

"And the very God of peace sanctify you wholly; and I pray God your whole spirit and soul and body be preserved blameless unto the coming of our Lord Jesus Christ" (1 Thessalonians 5:23).

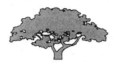

Symbol of The Tree of Life

God Created the Spirit, Soul and Body

𝕴n the beginning God fashioned the body of man and wrote of it in His Book of Life. David expressed this in one of his Psalms as he spoke to the Lord:

> *"For thou hast possessed my reins: thou hast covered me in my mother's womb. I will praise thee; for **I am fearfully and wonderfully made**: marvellous are thy works; and that my soul knoweth right well. My substance was not hid from thee, when I was made in secret, and curiously wrought in the lowest parts of the earth. Thine eyes did see my substance, yet being unperfect; and in thy **book all my members were written**, which in continuance were fashioned, when as yet there was none of them"* (Psalm 139:13-16).

"The supreme importance of the body is shown by the fact that God, the Architect, drew a plan which contained the various parts of the body–bones, muscles, nerves, blood vessels, tissues and organs. This book [Book of Life] which contains the plan is another of those wonderful volumes to be found in God's library. We shall be studying these books throughout eternity."[23]

God, having created the spirit, soul and body of man, is interested in everything that concerns these three parts. If there is any difficulty arising to affect this creature of His, *Yehovah Yireh* ("Provider-Lord"), will take care of it according to faith for He is the **Healer** (*Yehovah Rapha*) of His tripartite creation.

We, along with David, the sweet singer of Israel, give thanks to God for all His benefits:

---

[23]Arthur I. Brown, *God and You,* p. 10.

*"Bless the LORD, O my **soul**: and all that is within me, bless his holy name. Bless the LORD, O my soul, and forget not all his benefits: Who forgiveth all thine iniquities; who **healeth all thy diseases;"** (Psalm 103:1-3).*

Notice in the above quote that David was encouraging his *soul* to bless the Lord for forgiving iniquities and healing all its (soul's) diseases. The natural healing is a symbol of the spiritual healing. *Yahweh Rapha* is able to heal the spiritual, moral corruption and diseases of the soul as well as of the body.

David called God "The Health of My Countenance." He desired that God's health from within would show in his face. The condition of the "inner man" shows up on the "outer man." David describes his *soul* as being "cast down" or depressed and this he didn't want to show on his face:

*"Why art thou cast down, O my **soul**? and why art thou disquieted within me? hope in God: for I shall yet praise him, who is the **health of my countenance**, and my God"* (Psalm 43:5).

God Promised Healing to Israel [24]

*"... If thou wilt diligently hearken to the voice of the LORD thy God, and wilt do that which is right in his sight, and wilt give ear to his commandments, and keep all his statutes, I will put **none of these diseases** upon thee, which I have brought upon the Egyptians: for I am* [Jehovah-Rapha] *the LORD that **healeth thee"** (Exodus 15:26).

"The word *rapha* appears nearly seventy times in the Old Testament or *T'nach*. It always carries the meaning 'to restore,' 'to heal,' 'to cure' or 'a physician.' It is used not only in the *physical* sense but also in the *moral* and *psychical* [soul-spirit] meaning."[25]

Thank God! He still heals today! He is the same miracle-working Lord. He is able to deliver from every power of the devil *now*. Our God has not changed His covenant or His Name!

Isaiah, the Jewish prophet, questions the healing of the Lord in the 53rd chapter of his book (verse 1): *"Who has believed our report? And to whom is the arm of the LORD revealed?"* This question is answered in the second part of the Bible (the New Covenant) after the Lord's "arm" was revealed through Messiah Yeshua (Jesus):

---

[24]The first three articles are also included in my *Jewish Faith and the New Covenant* under "Tetragram," *Yahweh Rapha*, "The Lord Who Heals."
[25]"Message to Israel" magazine. October/November/December 1985. Article by A.J. Overton, Jr. *The Names of God*, a series: *Jehovah-Rapha*, p. 4.

"But though he had done so many miracles before them, yet they believed not on him: That the saying of Esaias [Isaiah] *the prophet might be fulfilled, which he spake, **Lord, who hath believed our report? and to whom hath the arm of the Lord been revealed?**"* (John 12:37-38).

Isaiah saw the suffering Messiah and exclaimed:

*"Surely he hath borne our sicknesses and carried our **pain**; but he was wounded for our transgressions, he was bruised for our iniquities, the chastisement of our peace was upon him; and by **his bruise** [singular case] **was healing granted unto us**"* (Isaiah 53:4-5, Isaac Leeser's translation).

We read of the fulfillment of this prophecy in the *Brit Hadasha*:

"When the even was come, they brought unto him [Yeshua] *many that were possessed with devils: and he cast out the spirits with his word, and **healed** all that were sick: That **it might be fulfilled** which was spoken by Esaias* [Isaiah] *the prophet, saying, **Himself took our infirmities, and bare our sicknesses**"* (Matthew 8:16-17).

David knew the Great Physician. His heart welled up in praise to Him as he spoke to his own soul: *"Bless the LORD, O my soul, and forget not all his benefits: Who forgiveth all thine iniquities; who **healeth all thy diseases;**"* (Psalm 103:2-3).

Moses knew the Great Physician. He was commanded by God to raise a brazen serpent upon a pole, so that the Israelites who had been poisoned *in their bodies*, looking upon it would *be healed!* Messiah declared that as Moses lifted up the serpent in the wilderness, so must the Son of Man be lifted up that those who were poisoned by sin and disease looking upon Him (that is, believing in Him) could be healed (John 3:14-15).

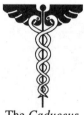

In the time of the Babylonian ruler Nimrod there was the worship of the serpent called *Aescalapius* which means "healer."[26] The heathen believed that this serpent entwined himself around a dead tree stump to bring renewed life to Nimrod. (The ancient pagans pictured Nimrod as the tree that had died.) The doctor's emblem today is a serpent entwined around a pole. It signifies healing.

The *Caduceus* emblem

---

[26]*Aescalapius* was the ancient Greek god of *medicine* that was made into the form of *one snake on a staff*. Some medical groups use the *Caduceus* (*two* snakes on a staff shown here) originally called the "wand of Hermes (Mercury)" which stood for *medicine* and for *commerce*.

"And the LORD said unto Moses, Make thee a fiery serpent, and set it upon a pole: and it shall come to pass, that every one that is bitten, when he looketh upon it, shall live. And Moses made a serpent of brass [copper], and put it upon a pole, and it came to pass, that if a serpent had bitten any man, when he beheld the serpent of brass [the antidote], he lived" (Numbers 21:8-9).

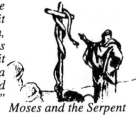
Moses and the Serpent

At the time of the first Passover, the Israelites were commanded to take a Lamb, kill it, shed its blood, and eat its meat. Not only was the blood given for redemption of the soul, but the meat of the lamb was to be eaten for strength and health for the journey into the Promised Land.

God expects every child of His who has applied the blood of the Lamb (Yeshua) to their hearts' door in faith for deliverance from soul bondage, to also partake, by faith, of the meat of that Lamb for strength and health through this wilderness (world) journey into the Promised Land! Not only was the blood of the Lamb shed for remission of our sins, but His body was bruised and broken for our *physical health*!

Yeshua was made a curse on a Tree of Death in order to redeem us from the curse of the law and so to have access to the Tree of Life. He who knew no sin was made sin so that we, believing upon Him, might be delivered from sin. He who knew no sickness, was made sick that we, believing on Him, might be delivered from sickness.

Lord of Health

O Lord of health and life,
What tongue can tell
How at thy touch
Were loosed the bands of hell,
How thy pure touch
Removed the leprous stain
And the polluted flesh
Grew clean again?
Yea, Lord we claim the promise of thy love,
Thy love, which can all guilt,
All pain remove;
Nigh to our souls
Thy great salvation bring.
Then sickness hath no pang,
And death no sting.
—G. Phillimore

Healing is ...

In the Atonement

"Surely he [Messiah] *hath borne our griefs* [sickness]*, and carried our sorrows: yet we did esteem him* [Messiah] *stricken, smitten of God, and afflicted. But he* [Messiah] *was wounded for our transgressions, he was bruised for our iniquities: the chastisement of our peace was upon him; and with his stripes we are healed"* (Isaiah 53:4-5).

"... and [Messiah] *healed all that were sick: That it might be fulfilled which was spoken by Esaias the prophet, saying, Himself took our infirmities, and bare our sicknesses"* (Matthew 8:16-17).

"Who his own self bare our sins in his [Messiah's] *own body on the tree, that we, being dead to sins, should live unto righteousness: by whose* [Messiah's] *stripes* [bruise] *ye were healed"* (1 Peter 2:24).

"Christ [Messiah] *hath redeemed us from the curse of the law, being made a curse for us: for it is written* [in the Old Testament, The T'nach], *Cursed is every one that hangeth on a tree:"* (Galatians 3:13, referring to Deuteronomy 21:22-23).

According to Deuteronomy 28:15-22, 27-29, and 35-61, *all sickness* and disease is a curse of the law. But, praise God, according to the Bible in Galatians 3:13 *Messiah* [Christ] *has redeemed us from the curse of the law!*

The Will of the Father

" ... for I am the LORD that healeth thee" (Exodus 15:26).

"And ye shall serve the LORD your God, and he shall bless thy bread, and thy water; and I will take sickness away from the midst of thee. There shall nothing cast their young, nor be barren, in thy land: the number of thy days I will fulfil" (Exodus 23:25-26).

"There shall no evil befall thee, neither shall any plague come nigh thy dwelling. With long life will I satisfy him, and show him my salvation" (Psalm 91:10, 16). [It has been known among my Jewish people, whenever the very religious are sick and they desire to be well, they will read Psalm 91 about three times or more as a sure remedy for their healing!]

"Bless the LORD, O my soul, and forget not all his benefits: Who forgiveth all thine iniquities; Who healeth all thy diseases" (Psalm 103:2-3). *"He sent his Word and healed them ... "* (Psalm 107:20).

$\mathbb{T}$ hrough Messiah Jesus

*"How God anointed Jesus of Nazareth with the Holy Ghost and with power: who went about doing good, and **healing** all that were **oppressed** of the devil; ..."* (Acts 10:38). [When God clothed Adam and Eve after their sin, their spirit, soul and body were covered. *Healing for man's **spirit**, **soul** and **body*** was provided by our wonderful Redeemer!]

*"And Jesus went about all the cities and villages, teaching in their synagogues, and preaching the gospel of the kingdom, and **healing** every **sickness** and every **disease** among the people"* (Matthew 9:35).

"And great multitudes came unto him [Messiah Jesus], *having with them those that were lame, blind, dumb, maimed, and many others, and cast them down at Jesus' feet; and he **healed** them: Insomuch that the multitude wondered, when they saw the dumb to speak, the maimed to be whole, the lame to walk, and the blind to see: and they glorified the God of Israel"* (Matthew 15:30-31).

$\mathbb{B}$ e Strong

A message connected to *healing* follows. It was my privilege to give this brief exhortation to the graduating class of SBC (Seattle Bible College) in June of 1980.

At the end of each year Jewish people recite a salutation to each other in Hebrew:

Hazak, hazak, vinit hazak–חֲזַק חֲזַק וּנִת חֲזַק (which means) *Be strong, be strong, and let us strengthen one another.* At the conclusion of some books of the *T'nakh* (the Hebrew Scriptures) this exhortation is found such as in *Kings,* the book of *Chronicles*, the books of *Jeremiah* and *Isaiah*, but they are hidden to most of us because they are *not translated!*

Then, at the conclusion of each of the books of Moses, there is only *one* word in *large Hebrew letters: **Hazak*** (be strong)! It also means "hold fast," "be of good courage," "be steadfast," "be strengthened." At the conclusion of *ten* other books of the Old Testament we also find this word ***Hazak** which is not translated.* (See for yourself in your Hebrew Bible the word חֲזַק, *Hazak!*)

We do find that this word *Hazak* is translated in the following verses:

"Be ye strong [hazak] therefore, and let not your hands be weak: for your work shall be rewarded" (2 Chronicles 15:7).

"Be strong [hazak] and of a good courage, fear not, nor be afraid of them: for the LORD thy God, he it is that doth go with thee; he will not fail thee, nor forsake thee" (Deuteronomy 31:6).

"Yet now be strong [hazak], O Zerubbabel, saith the LORD; and be strong [hazak], O Joshua, son of Josedech, the high priest; and be strong [hazak], all ye people of the land, saith the LORD, and work: for I am with you, saith the LORD of hosts:" (Haggai 2:4).

"Have not I commanded thee? Be strong [hazak] and of a good courage; be not afraid, neither be thou dismayed: for the LORD thy God is with thee whithersoever thou goest" (Joshua 1:9).

"Strengthen [hazak] ye the weak hands, and confirm the feeble knees. Say to them that are of a fearful heart, Be strong [hazak], fear not: ..." (Isaiah 35:3-4).

In the Hebrew NT:

"Thou therefore, my son, be strong [hazak] in the grace that is in Christ Jesus" (2 Timothy 2:1).

My exhortation to you, graduating class of 1980, is:

חזק *– Hazak! Be Strong!*

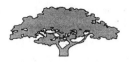

Healing of the Nations

*"... and the leaves of the tree were for the **healing** of the **nations**"* (Revelation 22:2).

We would do well to compare this with Revelation 21:4:

*"And God shall wipe away all tears from their eyes; and there shall be no more death, neither sorrow, nor crying, neither shall there be any more **pain**: for the former things [of the earth] are passed away."*

The Bible tells us that when the redeemed people of the Lord are "caught away" to be with Him, their *earthly* bodies will be transformed to that of the *heavenly*. They will be made like *His* glorious body which suffers no pain or sickness, sheds no tears of grief or sorrow, and experiences no death. We have already partaken of the "leaves of the Tree" for our healing *when we were on earth*; but there is no need for this when we are changed into the Lord's likeness (1 John 3:2). The *nations* who come to that Tree are the "earthly" people during the Millennium who will need to be healed from their sicknesses, etc.

How to Stay Healthy

by A.B. Simpson

Spiritual conditions are inseparably connected with our physical life. The flow of the divine currents may be interrupted by a little clot of blood; the vital current may leak out through a trifling wound.

If you want to keep physically healthy, keep from all spiritual sores, from all heart wounds and irritations.

One hour of fretting will wear out more vitality than a week of work; and one minute of malignity or ranking jealousy and envy will hurt more than a drink of poison!

Sweetness of spirit and joyousness of heart are essential to full health. Quietness of spirit, gentleness, tranquillity and the peace of God that passes all understanding are worth all the sleeping draughts in the country.

We do not wonder that some people have poor health when we hear them talk for half an hour. They have enough dislikes, prejudices, doubts and fears to exhaust the strongest constitutions.

Beloved, if you would keep your God-given life and strength, keep out of the things that would kill it. Keep it for Him and for His work, and you will find enough and to spare. STAY HEALTHY!

How Thought Controls Well-Being

by Wilfred Kent in *Conviction* Magazine

It is possible to so control and conduct your life, that you live with a positive sense of expectation, purpose and vitality. This should be the norm for your life. Yet, some may see this as a naive or vain hope. Sadly, those who do, live far below their potential.

It is a generally accepted scientific fact that one's physical condition is largely determined by his **emotions**. It is also true that one's emotional responses are regulated by the way he *thinks*. Thinking regulates feelings, and feelings govern health. **Formula**: *Thinking equals Emotions. Emotions equals Well-being.* When one thinks of painful or unpleasant thoughts, this in turn affects well-being.

I once met a man who was a perfect example of the above. He had suffered grave reversals. His wife died, his business went into bankruptcy, his friends abandoned him and his peers criticized him bitterly. Despite this, I found him indomitable, full of energy and eagerly planning the future. His face reflected a peace and confidence. It was a genuine pleasure to be in his presence.

When asked how it was that he could maintain such a healthy outlook on life, he replied: "I never worry! God is sovereign. It is He who gives and He who takes away. I have complete trust in Him. I reject all self-pity. I hold no grudges. I resist all painful memories and destructive thinking. But most importantly, I refuse to worry!" I was enriched by this man's faith.

Of all the areas about which we worry, the following statistics are true:

40% will never happen.
30% is passed and cannot be changed.
12% is petty.
10% is related to health.
8% is based on reality.

92% of our concerns are expended on unnecessary worry! How productive could we become if this energy could be channeled into more purposeful areas of our life? This is what the Apostle Paul encourages:

*"Don't worry over anything whatever: tell God every detail of your needs in earnest and thankful prayer, and the peace of God, which transcends human understanding, will keep constant guard over your hearts and minds as they rest in Jesus Christ ... **fix your mind on whatever is true and honorable and just and pure and lovely and praiseworthy** ... and you will find that the God of peace will be with you"* (Philippians 4:6-9, ARV).

What are you going to do to bring about happiness and well-being in your life ... for today?

—Wilfred Kent

Worry affects the circulation, the heart, the glands, the whole nervous system, and profoundly affects the health ... I have never known a man who died from overwork, but many who died from doubt!

—Dr. Charles Mayo of the Mayo Clinic

Discouragement, the Devil's Tool

Satan, realizing his time was short, decided to sell his tools and convert them to cash—much as many of his disciples are doing today.

At the sale were his old buddies: atheists, agnostics, and pragmatists. Each one was hoping to get back in business for a time—the time necessary to dispose at a profit to the coming generation.

Each tool was displayed in a way that would highlight its most effective use.

Among them were the Torch of Anger, the Knife of Malice, the Poison of Bitterness, the Idol of Pride, the Dagger of Deceit, the Hammer of Envy, the Club of Hate, the Goad of Disobedience, the Mask of Guile, and a host of others, each with its own price.

Surprisingly enough, sales were not brisk, the prices so high, and no one was buying much.

Still, most of the old bunch were hanging around hoping for a private tip on how to double their money.

Finally conversation developed when someone in the back saw a beat-up old tool with no price—a Wedge, labeled "Discouragement."

He asked, "Why, no price?" The devil answered: "Well, that's truly my very best tool. Look how I've used it. With the Wedge of Discouragement I can pry into a man's conscience when all the others are failing."

"Yes, I'll consider an offer." "But why is it so valuable?"

"Because I've used it all these years - and no one in this world seems to have found out I am its owner!"[27]

Effect of Thought in Health and the Body

by a non-Christian, James Allen

The body is the servant of the mind. It obeys the operations of the mind, whether they be deliberately chosen or automatically expressed. At the bidding of unlawful thoughts, the body sinks rapidly into disease and decay; at the command of glad and beautiful thoughts it becomes clothed with youthfulness and beauty.

Disease and health, like circumstances, are rooted in thought. Sickly thoughts will express themselves through a sickly body. Thoughts of fear have been known to kill a man as speedily as a bullet, and they are continually killing thousands of people just as surely though less rapidly. The people who live in fear of disease are the people who get it. Anxiety quickly demoralizes the whole body, and lays it open to the entrance of disease; while impure thoughts, even if not physically indulged, will soon shatter the nervous system.

Strong, pure, and happy thoughts build up the body in vigour and grace. The body is a delicate and plastic instrument, which responds readily to the thoughts by which it is impressed, and habits of thought will produce their own effects, good or bad, upon it.

Men will continue to have impure and poisoned blood so long as they propagate unclean thoughts. Out of a clean heart comes a clean life and a clean body. Out of a defiled mind proceeds a defiled life and corrupt body. Thought is the fount of action, life, and manifestation; make the fountain pure, and all will be pure.

Change of diet will not help a man who will not change his thoughts. When a man makes his thoughts pure, he no longer desires impure food.

---

[27]Written by an 85-year young Monk of Westminster Abbey, Mission City, British Columbia.

Clean thoughts make clean habits. The so-called saint who does not wash his body is not a saint. He who has strengthened and purified his thoughts does not need to consider the malevolent microbe.

If you would perfect your body, guard your mind. If you would renew your body, beautify your mind. Thoughts of malice, envy, disappointment, despondency, rob the body of its health and grace. A sour face does not come by chance; it is made by sour thoughts. Wrinkles that mar are drawn by folly, passion, pride.

As you cannot have a sweet and wholesome abode unless you admit the air and sunshine freely into your rooms, so a strong body and a bright, happy, or serene countenance can only result from the free admittance into the mind of thoughts of joy and goodwill and serenity.

On the faces of the aged there are wrinkles made by sympathy; others by strong and pure thought, and others are carved by passion: who cannot distinguish them? With those who have lived righteously, age is calm, peaceful, and softly mellowed, like the setting sun. I have recently seen a philosopher on his death-bed. He was not old except in years. He died so sweetly and peacefully as he had lived.

There is no physician like cheerful thought for dissipating the ills of the body; there is no comforter to compare with goodwill for dispersing the shadows of grief and sorrow. To live continually in thoughts of ill-will, cynicism, suspicion, and envy, is to be confined in a selfmade prisonhole. But to think well of all, to be cheerful with all, to patiently learn to find the good in all—such unselfish thoughts are the very portals of heaven; and to dwell day by day in thoughts of peace toward every creature will bring abounding peace to their possessor.

Good Health Department

In order for people to have good health they must control their temper. Anger has been proven to fill the body with poison, detrimental to health as well as piety. We cannot serve our heavenly Father well, unless we possess healthy bodies, neither can we prosper. It is the Father's will that we "prosper and be in health" (3 John 1:2).

Hatred, variance, wrath, strife, envy and all such destroy our bodily resisting powers and bring diseases and death.

"Then put to death those parts of you which belong to the earth—fornication, indecency, lust, foul cravings ... But now you yourselves must lay aside all anger, passion, malice ... now that you have

discarded the old nature with its deeds ..." (Colossians 3:5-9, New English Bible).

"As God required physical circumcision of the Jew, so today He requires of us 'Christ's way of circumcision,' which means 'being divested of the lower nature' with its emotions of 'anger, passion, malice' and self-centeredness. Such circumcision and such riddance of unlovely emotions are *clearly recognized by modern psychiatrists as causes or aggravations of the majority of all diseases.*"[28]

"Carnal emotions produce stress–which some authorities are now questioning as being the cause of all disease."[29]

"If you forgive not men their trespasses, neither will your Father in heaven forgive yours" is the teaching of the Master, and we cannot allow any of the above with malice, or thoughts of vengeance to be harbored in our mind, if we wish to have **good health** and long life. Evil thoughts will come. This is the devil's business, but we cannot permit them to linger with us. "You cannot prevent the birds from flying over your head, but you can keep them from building nests in your hair."

Ask the Lord, in the name of our Savior, to give you victory over your mind, and power only to retain good thoughts. Seek Him for wisdom daily, that you will know what is good wholesome food, and to enable you to control your appetite, and avoid over-eating. People usually eat all of the common food they relish, and then allow their appetite to be tempted by more tasty food at the end which they do not really need. It is the custom in many places to eat the desert first, and finish off on common food, which is wise.

Food From the Bible

𝕴n a first-time effort, *Neot Kedumim* (a nature resort in Israel) recently served a group of 280 Christian visitors from the U.S. a "biblical meal," each item on the menu based on a scriptural verse.

The dishes included *brown lentil stew,* (*"Then Jacob gave Esau bread and lentil stew ..."* (Genesis 25:34); *pita bread* (Elijah) *... looked around and there ... was a cake* [of bread] *baked over hot coals"* (1 Kings 19:16); *vegetables (*"Better a meal of vegetables where there is love than a fattened calf where is hate."* (Proverbs 15:17); and

---

[28]S.I. McMillen, *None of These Diseases*, pp. 21-22.
[29]J.D. Ratcliff, *Stress the Cause of All Disease?*, Reader's Digest, January, 1955.

labaneh, a tangy *milk* product.(*"... in a princely bowl she* [Yael] *brought him* [Sisera] *milk* [curds]" (Judges 5:25).

Healing in the Atonement

by F.F. Bosworth

THE INNER MAN	THE OUTER MAN
Adam, by his fall, brought sin into our *souls*.	Adam, by his fall, brought disease into our *bodies*.
Sin is therefore the work of the devil.	Disease is therefore the work of the devil. Jesus went about doing good, and healing all that were oppressed of the devil.
Jesus was "manifested to destroy the works of the devil" in the *soul*.	Jesus was "manifested to destroy the works of the devil" in the *body*.
The redemptive name "Jehovah Tsidkenu" reveals his redemptive provision for our *souls*.	The redemptive name "Jehovah Rapha" reveals his redemptive provision for our *bodies*.
On Calvary Jesus "bare our *sins*."	On Calvary Jesus bare our sicknesses.
He was made "sin for us" (2 Corinthians 5:21) when He "bare our sins" (1 Peter 2:24).	He was "made a curse for us" (Galatians 3:13) when he "bare our sicknesses" (Matthew 8:17).
"who his own self bare our sins in his body on the tree."	"by whose stripes ye were healed."
"who forgiveth all thine iniquities."	"who healeth all thy diseases."
"for ye are bought with a price: therefore glorify God in your ... spirit and ..."	"... in your body" (1 Corinthians 6:20).
The *spirit* is bought with a price.	The *body* is bought with a price.
Is remaining in sin the way to glorify God in your spirit?	Is remaining sick the way to glorify God in your body?
Since he "bare our sins," how many must it be God's will to save, when they come to Him? "whosoever believeth."	Since He "bare our sicknesses" how many must it be God's will to heal, when they come to Him? "He healed them all."
As God "made him to be sin for us who knew no sin ..."	"So God made Him to be sick for us who knew no sickness."

"since our substitute bore our sins, did he not do so that we might not bare them?"

"Christ bore our sins that we might be delivered from them. not sympathy, a suffering with, but substitution, a suffering for."

In the Lord's supper the wine is taken in remembrance of His death for our *souls* (1 Corinthians 11:25).

As many as received Him were born of God (John 1:12-13.

since our substitute bore our sicknesses, did he not do so that we might not bare them?

Christ bore our sicknesses that we might be delivered from them, not sympathy, a suffering with, but substitution, a suffering for."

In the Lord's supper the bread is eaten "in remembrance" of His death for our *bodies* (1 Corinthians 11:23-24).

As many as touched Him were made whole" (Mark 6:56).

Prayer for a Sick One

" ... *he whom thou* [Jesus] *lovest, is sick* (John 11:3).

You have taken a sick one to Jesus in prayer. Did you do so in this way, or did you say, 'My child, the one *I* love, is sick and I am anxious about him'? Did you forget Jesus' love for your dear one, that His anxiety was greater than yours could be? Did you think of your loved one as being even more truly HIS loved one? If in all our prayers to Him, His thought and care for us, and His interest in us, were uppermost instead of our own, how it would increase our faith and trust, and give peace and confidence in the issue!"[30]

---

[30]Rebecca Ruter Springer, *Intra Muros*.

Section 2
The Tongue

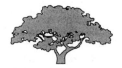

Three Diseases of the Tongue

by J.P. McCamey

Doctors are able to diagnose various diseases by examining the tongue. In the spiritual sense this is also true. *"And the tongue is a fire, a world of iniquity: so is the tongue among our members, that it defileth the whole body, and setteth on fire the course of nature; and it is set on fire of hell"* (James 3:6). There are several ways our tongues can defile us.

Gossip

Like a snake, gossip strikes without warning; and a reputation is dead. A suicide pinned to her coat a note that read simply, "They said." Many hear a story and instead of "in one ear and out the other," it is "in both ears and out the mouth!"

Some will protest, "But I only repeated the truth!" We can be very unchristian by helping spread a bad report on another. During a war a person with classified information could endanger others by telling all he knows, even though it is the truth. He can be shot as a traitor! We as Christian soldiers must not help spread stories, even though true, that help destroy another.

Cursing

Many develop a habit of cursing till it fills all conversation. A young boy was asked by his mother about his father's loss of temper. "Tell me what he said, but leave out the curse words!"

The boy answered, "Mom, if I leave out the curse words, I guess he didn't say anything!"

Some say it doesn't bother them to swear. A missionary pointed out a leper with toes rotted off. A friend asked, "Isn't the pain terrific?"

The missionary answered, "Not at this stage; the disease has gone too far."

One can curse long enough in his lifetime till irreverence becomes common. Others say, "I didn't mean anything by that burst of temper!" One answered that excuse by saying, "Don't say that. Look!" He then filled a glass to the brim with water, set it on a table, and struck the table next to the glass. Water splashed out. "Notice," he said. "Nothing splashed out of the glass but what was already in it!"

Your speech discloses the spiritual disease of the tongue! Jesus said, *"O generation of vipers, how can ye, being evil, speak good things? for out of the abundance of the heart the mouth speaketh"* (Matthew 12:34).

Lying

This habit of the tongue can also last a lifetime and eventually destroy conscience pangs. Someone said about a mutual friend: "He's lying at death's door." Another answered, "Yes, and it's a shame he's at death's door and still lying–still saying he has no need of God–when he knows better!"

James said: *"But the tongue can no man tame"* (James 3:8). We cannot easily change these defiling habits of the tongue just by willpower. The best way to conquer them is to receive Holy Spirit power! As the Spirit takes control and we speak in tongues, we then have supernatural help! This initial physical sign of the Holy Spirit's infilling is so appropriate in showing us He now has control. Read the Book of Acts and receive the power of the Holy Spirit that you may be delivered from the diseases of the tongue!

Symbol of the Holy Spirit

–*Pentecostal Evangel*

Healing by the Tongue

(When I was an Instructor at Seattle Bible College I gave the following message on *healing* in Chapel, January, 1984.)

The Contrary and Consecrated Tongue
Leshon Ha-Ra (The Evil Tongue)
Leshon Ha-Kodesh (The Sanctified Tongue)

One instance where "Leshon Ha-Ra" ("the tongue of evil") is found is in Leviticus 19:16 ("*You shall not go up and down as a slanderer among your people.*") Rabbis say that slander, talebearing, and evil talk are worse than the three cardinal sins of murder, immorality, and idolatry. Over and over again in the Book of Instructions (the Bible) we are warned that if we misuse our tongues, which God gave us to glorify Him, we shall be sick (see Proverbs 13:3).

"And Miriam and Aaron **spake against** *Moses because of the Ethiopian woman whom he had married: ..."* (Numbers 12:1).

We learn in the order of events after this that God called Moses, Aaron and Miriam to the Tabernacle of the Congregation and spoke to them about this *sin of the tongue.* He asked *"Were ye not afraid to* **speak against** *my servant Moses?"* God then departed from them and Miriam became leprous. She was mentioned first in the "speaking against" as if to imply that she was instrumental in swaying Aaron to agree with her in this sin. Aaron confesses their sin of evil speaking and Moses intercedes for Miriam's healing. Miriam was shut out from the camp for seven days after which she was brought back healed. The people did not journey on until first Miriam was brought in again.

Do you not see that the *tongue* affected Miriam's physical and spiritual *health?* According to the Jewish disciple, James, the tongue is an unruly member and it sets on fire the whole course of our natural bodies (James 3:6-10). How very true! Doctors have discovered that the digestion is affected, nerves burn, the brain is inflamed by a word of temper or of anger. The tongue speaks that which is within. Words of envy, fault-finding, complaining, resentment will affect the body. "Speaking against," in the case of Miriam, was a sin which was manifested in leprosy, affecting every member of her body. "Death and life are in the power of the tongue," the Word of God tells us. Also there is suffering and destruction as well as health in this little organ of our mouth: *"There is that speaketh like the piercings of a sword: but the tongue of the wise is* **health"** (Proverbs 12:18). Miriam criticized her brother Moses. Her *tongue* was the cause of her leprosy. It brought disease with the sentence of death.

Notice: Miriam didn't say anything false about Moses or criticize him for any sin. She spoke only that of which she did not approve. God calls this "speaking against." The greater part of speaking against is either from habit of criticism or from wrong motives.

Miriam was not the only one affected by her unruly member but also the body of God's people. They were delayed in the progress of their journey seven days because of Miriam's transgression of the tongue. One person's evil speaking–the wrong use of this little member–can affect the whole local body of God's people or the body to which that member is related.

On another occasion Israel murmured against Moses and Aaron in connection with the rebellion of Korah and Abiram and because of this use of their tongues in murmurings, disease was sent among them in judgment and 14,700 people died. When Aaron made atonement for the people, the disease was halted.

The Word of God says that the tongue is full of deadly poison (James 3:8). In Numbers 21:5-6 we see this poison experienced by the Israelites in the wilderness. God's people, redeemed from Egypt, saw the miracles of God, experienced His blessings—yet their tongues were full of deadly poison. They murmured and complained against their God.

What was the result of their evil speaking? It affected their physical bodies. The poison of the serpents was injected into their blood stream and their bodies began to swell. Much of the people died as a result. *Doctors know that that which poisons the mind, also poisons the blood and produces various forms of disease.* There is death and life in the power of the tongue. This poisonous tongue affected *all* of God's people. It, no doubt, was started by *one* member of their group. Not only do we poison ourselves with this unruly member but by the wrong use of our tongues we bring others into condemnation.

Praise God, there is a remedy of healing for the "contrary" tongue and it can become a "consecrated" tongue. What was the beginning of healing for the criticizing tongue of Miriam? First of all, confession of that sin, then the sanctified and consecrated tongue of Moses who interceded on her behalf and she was healed. What was the beginning of healing for the poisonous, murmuring tongues of the Israelites? First of all, a confession of that sin, and then the sanctified, consecrated tongue of Moses who interceded on their behalf. And this is the same procedure today!

Moses did not criticize Miriam nor condemn her, though she spoke against him; he simply interceded for her. Moses did not condemn the Children of Israel but simply interceded for them. This is (*Leshon haKodesh*) a consecrated tongue, a sanctified, controlled tongue!

The Holy Spirit through James said that no man can tame this little member of the body (James 3:6-8). No *man* can, but the Holy Spirit can control it if we turn it over to Him. He enables us to do that which we cannot do without Him! Do you want your tongue to be tamed—to be delivered—to be controlled—to be a consecrated tongue? Be filled with God's Holy Spirit, the Dove of Peace and Love!

–End of Message

Interesting Note: Not only is the tongue of *man* used in the case of healing but also the tongue of a *dog*! Healing qualities are found in both.

Archaeologists discovered in their excavations located in the area of Ashkelon (1991) that there were many dog burials related to the worship of the Phoenician *healing deities* Eshmoun and Resheph-Mukol. Perhaps because of the *curative powers* exhibited by dogs licking their sores and wounds, these animals were associated with *healing* in the ancient Near East. Their tongues held healing properties.[31]

We notice the story told by Messiah about the experience of the beggar Lazarus who lay at the rich man's gate full of sores (Luke 16:19-21). The rich man ignored the beggar (as everyone did) but the dogs *licked his sores*. Thus the dogs were more compassionate toward him than anyone. They were healing him with their tongues!

What the Tongue Can Do

The tongue can sin .... Psalm 39:1
The tongue can be kind .... Proverbs 10:21
The tongue can be healthy .... Proverbs 15:4
The tongue can be controlled (by the Spirit) .... James 1:26
The tongue can edify;
    It also can minister grace to others .... Ephesians 4:29
The tongue can produce a good, long life ..... Psalm 34:12-13
                         (See with 1 Peter 3:10.)

The Kind and Tender Word

by Duncan McNeil

God make me kind;
    So many hearts are breaking
    And many more are aching
    To hear the *tender word*.
    God make me kind;
    For I, myself am learning
    That my sad heart is yearning
    For some sweet word to heal my hurt.
    O Lord; do make me kind.
    God make me kind;
    So many hearts are needing

---

[31]Information from *Biblical Archaeology Review,* 1997.

The balm to stop the bleeding
That my *kind words* can bring.
God make me kind;
For I am also seeking
The cure in someone's keeping
They should impart to my sick heart
O Lord; do make me kind.
God make me kind;
So many hearts are lonely
And asking for this only -
The kind and tender word.
God make me kind;
To all who mutely ask it
Before they fill the casket
Or bouquets may be wreaths someday.
O Lord, do make me kind.

Sin of the Tongue

The Sin No One Confesses

by J. Stephen Conn

Almost every sin imaginable has been confessed to me during the more than two decades I have been a minister: stealing, lying, adultery, homosexuality, even murder. But I do not recall that anyone has ever confessed to me *the sin of gossip*. Yet gossip is surely one of the most prevalent of all sins, and one of those most severely condemned by God.

Perhaps one reason so few people feel guilty of telling about another person's faults is because we have developed clever ways to disguise what we are doing. Much of the worst slander is prefaced with a disclaimer such as, "I don't mean to be spreading rumors, but ..." That is an absurd statement. Anyone who makes it should immediately shut up or at least change the subject.

Gossip can be disguised as false sympathy: "Isn't it too bad how Joe beats his wife." Some gossip is passed off as a prayer request: "Now I'm just telling you this so you can pray about it." Then there is the person who pretends to ask an innocent question: "Is it true that George and Alice are getting a divorce?"

We also gossip by listening. If the receiver of stolen goods is as guilty as the thief, then is not the person who provides *a willing ear* the accomplice of the one who bears the tale? I consider it an insult when a person brings me gossip. In so doing he is passing judgment on me, assuming I delight in hearing such slander.

A gossip may argue, "But I am only telling the truth." The fact that a slanderous story is true does not necessarily justify its being told. If one man sins and another tells about it, the talebearer may have committed the *worst* sin of the two! For example, Genesis 9 tells how Noah became intoxicated and lay naked in his tent. It's a shame for anyone to get drunk–especially a preacher.

Noah's son Ham discovered his father's drunkenness and couldn't wait to go tell his two brothers about their old man. *All he told was the truth.* But Shem and Japheth refused to look upon their father's sin; instead *they covered him.* The sons who would not listen to or spread the gossip were blessed and they prospered. Ham, because of his gossip, was cursed and condemned to a life of servitude. Like all sinners who repent, Noah was forgiven. In the New Testament he is listed in Hebrews 11 as one of the great men of faith and righteousness.

In this scenario God's judgment against one who gossips was even more severe than it was against the man guilty of drunkenness and indecent exposure. That's something to think about the next time you hear yourself say: "I don't mean to gossip, but ...".

The Living Bible says: "Anyone who says he is a Christian but doesn't control his sharp tongue is just fooling himself, and his religion isn't worth much" (James 1:26).[32]

Description of the Tongue

Someone has said that *"The most ferocious monster in the world has his den just behind the teeth."* And Doctor Russell Bradley Jones reminds us that what Martin Luther called "that little flesh between the jaws" is a "concealed and dangerous weapon."

One of the first things a doctor suggests to a person who has come to him for a diagnosis of his sickness is to "stick out your tongue." From the appearance on it the doctor knows whether or not the patient has a disease. God, our great Physician, reads the heart by the tongue. "For out of the abundance of the *heart*, the mouth speaketh" (James 3:5).

---

[32]*Pentecostal Evangel,* November 12, 1989.

The Sin of Backbiting

"LORD who shall abide in thy tabernacle? who shall dwell in thy holy hill? ***He that backbiteth not with his tongue,*** *..."* (Psalm 15:1, 3).

What is *backbiting?* All a man says may be true as the Bible but it is evil speaking of a person who is absent; relating something evil which was really done or said by one who is not present when it is related. He is not there to answer for himself. Backbiting is anything said about an absent person, whether true or untrue, that in any way reflects on his moral or spiritual character. If the thing you have to say will in the least degree lower the one talked about in the estimation of the one to whom you are telling it, then you are about to commit the *sin* of backbiting, and for the sake of your own precious immortal soul as well as that of the other party and the cause of Christ in general, refrain from saying it, because truly *"death and life are in the power of the tongue."*

As the above Scripture tells: the backbiter will not dwell in God's Holy Hill. He may profess all that he pleases, but, if he be a backbiter, he will be numbered with the other workers of iniquity and will receive his just reward, except *he repent now.* Backbiters are classed with *murderers, thieves, whoremongers, etc.* God will mete out His judgment accordingly. No *excuse* will be accepted of the Lord in His day of *judgment.* Those who are guilty of this evil will hear the same words as the murderer, thief, and whoremonger. *"Depart from me ye workers of iniquity"* (Matthew 7:23). *Only those who have deeply repented of it, forsaken it, and have it covered with the atoning blood of Jesus* ***will escape the judgment.***

Is the sin of backbiting (so despised by the Lord), treated as such a light matter that the backbiter should be allowed to continue to spread his poison and remain a member of the assembly without being dealt with? May God in Heaven help us to raise the *standard* against this thing, probably, the *worst of all evils.* May God help us properly classify it and to place the *backbiter where he belongs.* Make him to see that the sin of *backbiting* is as great a sin as *murder, adultery* or *stealing* and to hold him to the same form of *repentance.*

In Paul's letter to the Romans he classifies *backbiting* and all that it means with *fornication, murder, and every evil work.*

"And even as they did not like to retain God in their knowledge, God gave them over to a reprobate mind, to do those things which are not convenient; Being filled with all unrighteousness, fornication, wickedness, covetousness, maliciousness; full of envy, murder, debate, deceit, malignity; **whisperers,** **Backbiters,** *haters of God,*

*despiteful, proud, boasters, inventors of evil things, disobedient to parents, Without understanding, covenantbreakers, without natural affection, implacable, **unmerciful**: Who knowing the judgment of God, that they which commit such things **are worthy of death**, not only do the same, but have pleasure in them that do them"* (Romans 1:28-32).

You will also see in Paul's writings to the Galatians that he throws them all in the same class and says, *"And they which do such things **shall not inherit the kingdom of God**"* (Galatians 5:19-21).

A.B. Simpson said: "I would rather play with forked lightning or take in my hands living wires, with their fiery currents, than speak a **reckless word** against any servant of Christ, or idly repeat the **slanderous darts** which thousands of Christians are hurling on others, to the hurt of their own souls and bodies."

"Speak evil of no man," says the great apostle–as plain a command as, "Thou shalt do no murder."

*"If any man among you seem to be religious, and **bridleth not his tongue**, but deceiveth his own heart, **this man's religion is vain**"* (James 1:26).

*"Moreover if thy brother shall trespass against thee, go and tell him his fault **between thee and him alone**: if he shall hear thee, thou hast gained thy brother"* (Matthew 18:15).

It gratifies our pride to relate those faults of others, of which we think ourselves not guilty! Two good mottoes to follow are: "Speak *after* others; never *against* others; always *well* of others." "Complain of nothing; neither of persons or of things."

"Judge not, that ye be not judged. For with what judgment ye judge, ye shall be judged: and with what measure ye mete, it shall be measured to you again. And why beholdest thou the mote that is in thy brother's eye, but considerest not the beam that is in thine own eye? Or how wilt thou say to thy brother, Let me pull out the mote out of thine eye; and, behold, a beam is in thine own eye? Thou hypocrite, first cast out the beam out of thine own eye; and then shalt thou see clearly to cast out the mote out of thy brother's eye" (Matthew 7:1-5).

The tongue of the gossiper is unclean. Gossip is trifling talk–talking about others' weaknesses, failures, peculiarities, etc. The literal meaning of the words "gossiper" and "tattler" is "bubbler." A gossiper and tattler simply cannot keep still. They are bubbling over with talk which is anything but profitable and proper. Whispering about another is a mark of hatred. Speaking against a person behind his back (back-biting) is one of the meanest things to which we can lend our lips. Proverbs 11:13 tells: *"A talebearer revealeth secrets: but he that is* *of a **faithful spirit** concealeth the matter." **"Love covereth all sins"*** (Proverbs 10:12). In other words when a sin is discovered in another the faithful spirit and love does not gossip about it but conceals and hides it–not excusing it–but a believer prays for that person's deliverance! Are we not to have compassion for that one who is bound? The Lord is moved with compassion when He sees the bondage of the sinner or of the one who believes in Him. So are we to be as priests of the Most High God–filled with that same compassion for we are ministers of reconciliation.

– Author unknown

The Sin of Spiritual Cannibalism

by Robert H. Farish

Spiritual cannibalism is, in the Galatian letter, put as the anti-thesis of the duty to "love thy neighbor as thyself."

*" ... Thou shalt love thy neighbour as thyself. But if ye **bite and devour** one another, take heed that ye be not consumed one of another"* (Galatians 5:14-15).

"Cannibalism" is defined as "eating human flesh by mankind or of any animal by its own kind." The revolting and unnatural action of cannibalism (biting and devouring one another) is selected by the Holy Spirit as a fit figure to describe the behavior of those members of the church whose actions toward one another can have only one result if persisted in, namely, mutual destruction.

When a member of the Lord's church bites and devours another member of the Lord's church, he is devouring his own kind. The very thought of physical cannibalism is revolting to any normal person. Visualize such a scene! A family of brothers and sisters eagerly gorging themselves on one another, biting out chunks of one another and gulping them down. Soon the inevitable destruction of that family occurs. Such is the picture painted by the Holy Spirit to deter members of the church from a course which will result in their being "consumed one of another."

The law regulating a Christian's action toward another Christian is: "Thou shalt love thy neighbor as thyself." The opposite course is introduced by the writer with the word "but." The preposition "but" expresses opposition, contradiction, or antithesis. "Spiritual cannibal-ism" is the antithesis of "love thy neighbor as thyself." The thesis upon which a Christian–any Christian–whether he be elder, preacher, editor, etc., must operate in his relation to a neighbor is, "Thou shalt love thy neighbor as thyself."

There is no acceptable synthesis between these two courses. They are contrary one to the other; never shall the two meet on divinely approved middle ground. The law is inexorable: "if ye bite and devour one another, take heed that ye be not consumed one of another." The consequences of "spiritual cannibalism" is mutual destruction. "God is no respecter of persons." He has licensed no one to bite and devour with impunity.

A dog fight may start off with only two dogs involved, but it will not long continue limited to just two, if there are other dogs around, for others will get into the act and a melee will develop in which all are involved. In like manner, when one brother "bites" another, the urge to retaliate in kind is strong in the one "bitten." The urge to "bite" the "biter" is the strength of this device of the devil. When the one whose good name has been ruthlessly injured gives way to the urge to bite back, others are drawn into a ghoulish orgy of spiritual cannibalism. If members of the church would be caused to see that successful "biting and devouring" is a victory for the forces of evil, perhaps the relish for such should abate.

How can "spiritual cannibalism" be avoided? The answer to this is given by the apostle. He wrote: *"But I say, walk by the Spirit, and ye shall not fulfill the lust of the flesh."* When one "bites and devours," he is fulfilling the lust of the flesh. There is no spiritual gratification to be derived from "spiritual cannibalism." The apostle then proceeds to list the works of the flesh. This list includes more sins which can be identified as "biting and devouring" than any other type. Enmities, strife, jealousies, wraths, factions, division, parties, envyings, are listed in the same catalogue with fornication; uncleanness, lasciviousness, drunkenness, etc. By what authority can a Christian condemn one but condone or tolerate the other?

The approved actions of reproving and rebuking are not to be confused with the condemned action of "biting and devouring." Every member of the church has the divinely imposed obligation to "reprove and rebuke"; he must also "contend earnestly for the faith which was once for all delivered to the saints"—but every member of the church is required to avoid "biting and devouring." There is no conflict between the divine requirement and the divine prohibition. The Holy Spirit requires the Christian to "reprove, rebuke and exhort with all longsuffering and teaching" (2 Timothy 4:2). The same Holy Spirit requires the Christian to refrain from "biting and devouring."

Care should be exercised to avoid arraying "truth" against "love." Mistakes are often made by quoting passages of Scripture *which approve rebuking a brother,* in *justification of actions* which by no stretch of the imagination can be identified as anything but "spiritual cannibalism." It is a serious blunder to seek to justify "biting and devouring" by quoting passages which require "reproving and rebuking." It is equally serious to condemn proper "reproving and rebuking" by citing prohibitions against "biting and devouring."[33]

Gossips

> A gossip speaks ill of all, and all of her.

> Believe not half you hear, repeat not half you believe; when you hear an evil report, halve it, then quarter it, and say nothing about the rest of it.

–Spurgeon

> To learn to speak several languages is easy; the difficulty is to learn to be silent in one!

> Language is the dress of thought; every time you talk, your mind is on parade.

> By examining the tongue of a patient, physicians find out the disease of the body, and philosophers the disease of the mind.

–Justin

The Backbiter and His Doom

by Marvin C. Miller

Be Wise

A wise old Owl sat up in an oak,
   The more he heard, the less he spoke;
   The less he spoke, the more he heard;
   Now! Wasn't he a wise old bird?

"LORD, who shall abide in thy tabernacle? who shall dwell in thy holy hill? He that walketh uprightly, and worketh righteousness, and speaketh the truth in his heart. He that backbiteth not with his tongue, nor doeth evil to his neighbour, nor taketh up a reproach against his neighbour" (Psalm 15:1-3).

All down through the ages the work of God has suffered; whole denominations have been split and divided; individual assemblies have been shattered and ruined; homes have been wrecked; hopes have been blasted, and lives have suffered irreparable damage as a result of the deadly sin of *backbiting*, which includes all that we know as talebearing, whispering, evil-speaking, defaming, sowing discord, bearing false witness, spreading false reports, and repeating gossip.

---

[33]*The C.E.I. Publishing Company,* Athens, Alabama.

This sin is so far-reaching and destructive in its effect, so easy to commit and so hard to get rid of, and so little has been done to throw it into the light of the scripture! A careful study of God's Word is worthy of our earnest consideration in order that we might shield ourselves against indulging in it, and from the wrath of God which is kindled against those who do indulge in it, and from the results that are sure to follow if indulged in.

In order that the Holy Spirit, to whom we must look for guidance, may bring the truth concerning the sin being dealt with, we must enter into the study with sincere hearts and open minds, willing to receive the Word of God as it deals with this awful, deadly, destructive sin. Prejudice and insincerity will hinder the truth from being revealed.

God's Word Concerning It

We shall be helped to refrain from this evil if we get a clear understanding of what God has to say concerning it. Our attention is called to the fact that the whole business of backbiting, evil-speaking, whispering, talebearing, etc., is distinctly forbidden. *"Thou shalt not go up and down a tale bearer among the people"* (Leviticus 19:16). Just as definite and just as positive as He is in His commandments, "Thou shalt not kill [murder], Thou shalt not steal, Thou shalt not commit adultery," so is He in this command. Whether the tale borne be true or false makes no difference, *Thou shalt not.*

God strictly forbids it and makes plain His hatred towards it, *"These six things doth the LORD hate: yea, seven are an abomination unto him: A proud look, a lying tongue, and hands that shed innocent blood, an heart that deviseth wicked imaginations, feet that be swift in running to mischief, a false witness that speaketh lies, and he that soweth discord among brethren"* (Proverbs 6:16-19).

The tale bearer will raise his eyebrows lightly, remark that he despises gossip, and will have nothing to do with it. "But *they say* that Mrs. So-and-So is losing out entirely spiritually, and I must say I don't wonder. *They say*, there is some mystery about her case, and the worst of it is, *they say*, her husband is getting wise to it all. *They say*, he looks awfully worried." And thus the *tale bearer* injects into the ears of his hearers all that *they say*. The truth of the whole thing may be that Mrs. So-and-So and her husband are undergoing a fiery trial and are broken and crushed before the Lord. Never are they more concerned about the things of the Lord and the affairs of one another. Heavy-hearted and broken in the trial their countenance reveals a change from the ordinary. The *evil surmiser* takes the opposite and begins the *"they say."*

The Tattler spreads his evil surmisings everywhere, stirring and arousing the suspicions of others. God in His high and holy place, having forbidden it, looks upon the **tale bearer** with **burning hatred**. And why does the wrath of God thus burn against the **tattler**? *"He soweth discord among the brethren."*

Be sure, *"Whatsoever a man soweth that shall he also reap."* If a man sows wheat, he reaps wheat. If he sows *discord*, he will reap *discord.* How happy Satan and his host must be as they watch the *tale bearer* go up and down among the brethren! From home to home, from person to person he goes, sowing his poisonous seed, until whole churches and whole communities have been covered! And when his seed springs up, *what a harvest!* Reputations are ruined; homes are wrecked; the work of God is marred; whole churches are split and filled with discord; chiefest of friends are hopelessly separated (Proverbs 16:12), and multitudes are left with broken and aching hearts all through life.

Oh, my brother, my sister, what could be more devilish than to SOW DISCORD AMONG THE BRETHREN? Is it any wonder that the wrath of God burns so against it? ... The evil of *backbiting* and all that it means has always been, is now, and always will be a menace to the church, home, society, virtue and reputation. So terrible and dreadful was it in the mind of Plautus, who lived centuries ago, that he said, "Those men who carry about and who listen to accusations should all be hanged, if, so it could be at my decision, the carriers by their tongue, the listeners by their ears." Savage, to say the least, is his suggestion, but hardly is it to be compared with the words of the Lord God Almighty when He said: *"These shall go away into everlasting punishment"* (Matthew 25:46). *"And the Lord shall cut him asunder and appoint him his portion with the hypocrites: there shall be weeping and gnashing of teeth"* (Matthew 24:51). ...

Backbiting has a triple blow, wounding him that commits it, him against whom it is committed, and the listener to it. Once the words of the backbiter are out, they go on and on unchecked. As an echo rings from mountain side to mountain side, so they ring back into the ears of the hearers. Just as a snowball increases in size as it rolls, so *slander* grows as it spreads. *Slander* is remembered long after good words are forgotten. ***Tale Bearers are as bad as Tale Makers.*** It is to be remembered that the bearer of the tale is as guilty as the maker of it. ... Those who live and walk in the Spirit and are led by the Spirit avoid bearing tales and also hearing them, but rather concealeth the matter for this is the way of the Spirit. If a man see another man's fault, and it is impossible for him to doubt the fault, and if he live, walk in, and be led of the Holy spirit, he will do as the Word of God declares he must do. *"If a man be overtaken in a fault, ye **which are**"* *spiritual, restore such an one **in the spirit of meekness;** considering thyself, lest thou also be tempted"* (Galatians 6:1) *"**speak evil of no man"*** (Titus 3:2). ... When we cannot truthfully speak well of another, we will do well to keep silence. If our church or community is endangered by another's fault, and we are sure of his fault, then let us deal with him according to the Scriptures as has been mentioned; and let it be remembered that *He **who speaks well of others is himself spoken of with respect!***

Slander, a Dangerous Weapon

by Oswald J. Smith

No Christian worker can take up the sword of slander and escape the consequences. *"All they that take the sword shall perish with the sword"* (Matthew 26:52). So spake Jesus, and history has repeatedly borne testimony to the truthfulness of His warning. Men who have slandered others have either been ruined by slander themselves or have been judged by God with death. And it makes no difference whatever, be it borne in mind, whether the slander is true or false–the result is the same.

Judgment is God's prerogative, not man's. His Word is *"Touch not mine anointed, and do my prophets no harm ..."* (Psalm 105:15). The statements made may be absolutely true, but since no mere man may capably judge, God's servants are accountable to Him and to Him alone. And woe betide the man who dares to set himself up as a judge and publicly slander his fellow-workers! God will not let it pass. ...

> *"Judge not, that ye be not judged, For with what ye judge, ye shall be judged: and with what measure ye mete, it shall be measured to you again. And why beholdest thou the mote that is in thy brother's eye, but considerest not the beam that is in thine own eye? or how wilt thou say to thy brother, Let me pull out the mote out of thine eye; and, behold, a beam is in thine own eye? Thou hypocrite, first cast out the beam out of thine own eye, and then shalt thou see clearly to cast out the mote out of thy brother's eye"* (Matthew 7:1-5).

Remember this, my friend: he who *slanders* is working with the *devil*. Satan is a *slanderer*. He is continually accusing us before God. That is his biggest job and his most destructive work. O my brother, are you going to do the *devil's work*? Are you letting him use you as one of his slanderers? One of the greatest evils that afflicts the world today is that of gossiping and talebearing. You find it everywhere you go. It is rife in the business world, in the office, and in the factory. Its evil influence has permeated every strata of society, from the palace to the slum, and it rears its ugly head in the Church as many Christians have known from painful experience. The *tongue* of the *gossiper* has destroyed empires and has cast down many mighty men. Ruined lives, blighted homes, broken hearts, and sundered friendships have been caused by the *talebearer* and through the chatter of *idle tongues*.

Too late, sometimes, people learn what harm has been wrought by giving too ready an ear to rumor and too ready a tongue to pass it on. *"Behold, how great a matter a little fire kindleth"* wrote the apostle, James (3:5) about the *tongue*. Nothing is more needed in this world today than the manifestation of the Spirit of Christ that will scorn to speak evil of another when no good purpose can possibly be accomplished. The flower of Christian character will never bloom in the atmosphere of slander and distraction.

May God help us always to live, think, act, and speak in the light of eternity! Then, instead of getting our eyes on man and judging him, watching for either his virtues or his faults, we will keep our eyes fixed on the Christ who indwells him and see no man save Jesus only.

*"If any man among you seem to be religious, and **bridleth not his tongue**, but deceiveth his own heart, **this man's religion is vain**"* (James 1:26).
–*Pilgrim Tract Society,* Inc. Randleman, N.C.

Stick Out Your Tongue

by Morris Chalfant

An aged saint once declared, "Some Christians are like an old shoe–all worn out but the tongue!"

When we fail to guard our lips, our conversation is sure to be filled with exaggeration, insinuation, and foolish prattling that does not glorify God. Our spiritual energy is consumed in a welter of words.

Two kinds of human beings talk too much–the masculine and the feminine.

Psychologists tell us that every sensation goes to some brain center where it is registered. If that is true, the speech center must be highly developed.

The tongue is the most overworked muscle in the body. There is this difference, however: an over-exercised arm tires you; *an over-worked tongue tires your friend!*

A young man was sent to Socrates to learn to be an orator. On being introduced to the philosopher, he talked so incessantly that Socrates asked for a double fee.

"But why are you charging me double?" asked the young fellow.

"Because," replied the great orator, "I see I must teach you two sciences–the one, how to hold your tongue; and the other, how to speak." And the first is generally more difficult.

If you are the average articulate person, according to one publisher, you will use 35,000 words each day. Each of us would fill the shelves of a college library if all of our words were written in books.

But it may be a good thing that all our words are not written down here on earth. How much of what we say each day is worth hearing again? How many of our words are uplifting, encouraging, helpful, instructive, beneficial? How many would be better left unsaid? Many problems in our world could be solved if men [and women] learned to *control their tongues*. [At this last sentence, Duane Bagaas, my son said: "Women are coy but men are obvious; both are cutting."]

It is said, "The spoon always seems twice as large when you have to take a dose of your own medicine." In the light of Jesus' teaching in Matthew 12 [verses 34-37], we might paraphrase that truth, "Words which appear to be just tiny molehills of idleness and frivolity here will loom as mountains of error when we face them in the judgment." Not only the wicked utterances of the tongue will rise up against us in that day, but for every foolish, idle word we shall also be called to give a strict account.

Solomon summarized the matter in Ecclesiastes 5:2: "Be not rash with thy mouth, and let not thine heart be hasty to utter any thing before God: for God is in heaven, and thou upon earth: therefore *let thy words be few*."

Charles H. Spurgeon was once visited by a woman who felt that his tie was too long. To her it was a sign of worldliness. Spurgeon listened patiently, took off the tie, handed it to the woman, and told her to adjust it to the length she thought it ought to be. "But," he added, "dear sister, may I perform a service for you too?"

"Certainly," she replied, "I shall appreciate it very much."

"Well," said Spurgeon, "you also have something which is too long to be in accord with Christian humility, which has caused me and others a great deal of grief. I should like to cut it down to its proper length."

"Indeed," she said, "what can it be? Here, use the scissors as you please."

"But the tongue can no man tame," James said. "It is an unruly evil, full of deadly poison. We use it to bless God, and we use it to curse men ... These things ought not so to be" (see James 3:8-10).

You can't control your words, but God can. The words that come out of your mouth reflect what is in your heart. To change your words, you must have your heart changed.

What you said today is recorded. You will hear those words again; and they will justify you or they will condemn you because they will reveal what is in your heart.

Ask God today to take out of your heart the root of those evil words and set a watch by your lips.

–Pentecostal Evangel, April 23, 1989, p.7

It is easy to make a mountain out of a molehill: all you do is add dirt.

–Back to the Bible Broadcast

The Power of the Tongue [34]

Keep a watch on your words, my brother,
      For words are wonderful things.
They are sweet, like the bees' fresh honey;
      Like the bees, they have terrible stings.
They can bless like the glad, warm sunshine,
      And brighten a lonely life.
They can cut in the strife of anger,
      Yes, like a two-edged knife.
Let them pass through your lips unchallenged
      If their errand be true and kind,
If they come to support the weary,
      To comfort and help the blind.
If a bitter, revengeful spirit
      Prompts the words, let them be unsaid.
They may pass through the brain like lightning,
      Or fall on the heart like lead.
Keep them back if they are cold or cruel,
      Under bar and lock and seal;
The wounds they make, my brother,
      Are always slow to heal.
May Christ guard your lips, and ever
      From the time of your early youth
May the words that you daily utter
      Be the words of the beautiful truth.
                              –Selected

---

[34]Excerpts from *The Serpent's Fang,* "The Cure For Evil Speaking" by S.L. Flowers, a booklet of 47 power-packed pages.

Talkativeness

Talkativeness is utterly ruinous to deep spirituality. The very life of our spirits passes out through our speech, and hence all superfluous talk is a waste of the vital forces of the heart. In fruit-growing it often happens that excessive blossoming prevents a good crop, and often prevents fruit altogether; and by so much loquacity the soul runs wild in word-bloom, and bears no fruit. I am not speaking of sinners nor of legitimate testimony for Jesus, but of that incessant loquacity of nominally Christian persons, and of professors of purifying grace. It is one of the greatest hindrances to deep, solid communion with God.

Notice how people will tell the same things over and over; how insignificant trifles are magnified by a world of words; how things that should be buried are dragged out into gossip; how a nonessential is argued and disputed over; how the solemn deep things of the Holy Spirit are rattled over in a light manner, until one who has the real baptism of divine silence in his heart feels he must unceremoniously tear himself away, and retire alone where he can gather up the fragments of his mind and rest in God, or his usefulness will be impaired. Not only do we need cleansing from sin, but our natural human spirit needs a radical death to its own voice, activity and wordiness.

See the evil effects of so much talk. First, it dissipates the spiritual power. The thought and feeling of the soul are like powder and steam-the more they are condensed, the greater their power. The steam, if properly compressed, would drive a train forty miles an hour; if allowed too much expanse would not move it an inch; and so true action of the heart, if expressed in a few Holy Ghost selected words, will sink into the mind to remain forever, but if dissipated in any rambling conversation is likely to be of no profit.

Second, talkativeness is a waste of valuable time. If the hours spent in useless conversation were spent in *secret prayer* or good reading, we would soon reach a region of soul life and divine peace, far beyond our present dreams.

Third, loquacity inevitably leads to saying unwise, unpleasant or harmful things. In religious conversation we soon churn up all the cream our souls have in them, and the rest of our talk is all pale skim milk, until we get alone with God and feed in His green pastures and the cream rises again. The Holy Spirit warns us that *in the multitude of words there wanteth not sin*. It is impossible for the best of saints to talk beyond a certain point without saying something unwise, or severe, or foolish, or erroneous.

We must settle this personally. If others are noisy and gabby, I must determine to live in constant quietness and humility of heart. I *must guard my speech* as a sentinel does a fortress, and with all respect for others, must many a time cease from conversation, or withdraw from company to enter into deep communion with my precious Lord.

The cure for loquacity must be from within; sometimes by an interior furnace of affliction and suffering that burns out the excessive effervescence of the mind, or by an overmastering revelation to the soul of the awful majesty of God and eternity, which puts an ever-lasting hush upon the natural faculties.

To walk in the Spirit, we must avoid talking for talk's sake, or merely to entertain. To speak effectively, we must speak in God's appointed time, and in harmony with His indwelling Holy Spirit. When we read the words of Jesus as recorded in Matthew 12:36, "But I say unto you, That every *idle* word that men shall speak, they shall give account thereof in the day of judgment," we begin to realize something of the importance of the subject before us and are made to cry with David, "Set a watch, O LORD, before my mouth; keep the door of my lips" (Psalm 141:3).

King Solomon must have had a few light, talkative people to deal with in his time. Here are a few of the pointed verses from the pen of this wise man. "Even a fool, when he holdeth his peace, is counted wise: and he that shutteth his lips is esteemed a man of understanding" (Proverbs 17:28). And, *"A fool's voice is known by **multitude of words"*** (Ecclesiastes 5:3).

The Early Church was no doubt burdened with them also, for James deals with loquacity with ungloved hands. *"If any man among you seem to be religious, and bridleth not his tongue"* (James 1:26). Solomon seems to boil the whole trouble down when he says, *"In the **multitude** of words there wanteth not sin"* (Proverbs 10:19).

Idle Words

*"That every **idle word** that men shall speak, they shall give account thereof in the day of judgment"* (Matthew 12: 36). There is no clearer index to one's heart condition than his words. The Bible statement, "As he *thinketh* in his heart, so is he," refers to the source, as it is in the mind these idle words have their rise. Words are simply convey-ances by which our thoughts are carried to others. Back of all our thoughts is the heart, the fountain, from which they spring.

"Out of the heart," Jesus said, "proceed evil thoughts," and the only way we have of passing them on to others is by word of mouth, if they are to be fully understood. We see the necessity, therefore, of having the fountain pure so that the thoughts proceeding from it, and reaching those about us, by means of our speech may also be pure and clean.

James asks the question, "Doth a fountain send forth at the same place sweet water and bitter? ... so can no fountain both yield salt water and fresh" (James 3:11-12). Our words are so certainly indicative of the soul's condition that Jesus tells us, "By thy words thou shalt be justified, and by thy words thou shalt be condemned" (Matthew 12:37).

One of the qualifications of a bishop in the days of Paul was, "Not doubletongued" (1 Timothy 3:8). Their wives also must be "not slanderers." It seems that a great deal of stress was *placed on a right* use of *the tongue* in those early days of the Christian Church. They evidently understood that an idler was a dangerous person to have among the brethren; so they forestalled this peril, at least in their leaders and their wives.

Idle words are not necessarily evil words, though they are apt to lead to evil. There is a danger of going to either extreme; and while the one leading to a free use of idle words is the greater evil because of the possible result, it is also possible to do harm by assuming a melancholy attitude. The religion of Jesus Christ is a joyful and cheerful religion, and a long face does not fit it very well.

By idle words we mean all light, frivolous, or foolish conversation from which no good can be expected–talk that we would not like to be engaged in when Jesus comes, talk that we would be ashamed to face at the bar of God. Any word or words that might lead to an unholy thought or desire, or result in evil of any kind, might properly be denominated idle words.

In 1 Peter 1: 15 we read, "Be ye holy in all manner of *conversation*." If we will follow this admonition, we will not go very far astray.

It was said of Him who was the Example in all things, "Christ also suffered for us, leaving us an example, that ye should follow his steps: who did no sin, *neither was guile* [deception] *found in his mouth*" (1 Peter 2:21-22).

It is not a difficult task to ascertain the spiritual condition of the average professor of religion. The same is true today as when the maid told Peter, as he stood by the fire warming himself, *"Thy speech bewrayeth* [betrayeth] *thee."* The heart that is filled with the love of God and overflowing with concern for lost humanity will not spend very much time in idle conversation.

We read in Psalm 34:12-13, *"What man is he that desireth life, and loveth many days, that he may see good? Keep thy tongue from evil, and thy lips from speaking guile* [deception]. Then in 1 Peter 3:10, we have a like passage, *"For he that will love life, and see good days, let him refrain his tongue from evil, and his lips that they speak no guile* [deception]."

"Death and life are in he power of the *tongue*" (Proverbs 18:21). "Suffer not thy mouth to cause thy flesh to sin; neither say thou before the angel, that it was an error: wherefore should God be angry at thy voice, and destroy the work of thine hands?" (Ecclesiastes. 5:6).

God takes account of all our words. He tells us that "our conversation is in heaven," and we will surely meet it all again. We have often wondered, if a book were written containing all our words, whether we would be willing to meet it at the judgment; be willing to have it opened up before the assembled millions when the world is on fire and the elements melting with fervent heat.

Unkind words, foolish words, malicious words, complaining words, insinuating words, all words that are not profitable to the speaker and the hearer, are idle words and will meet us at the bar of God to condemn and destroy. How careful, then, we should be of our conversation and see to it that we say nothing that will condemn us on that last, great day!

–End of message on *The Power of the Tongue*

The Tongue–Good and Bad

Xanthus, a Greek philosopher was entertaining some friends at dinner. For the occasion he told his servant to serve the best thing he could find in the market. The resultant menu consisted of several courses of tongue cooked in various ways. Angry with his servant Xanthus asked, "Did I not tell you to get the best thing in the market?" Said the servant, "I did get the best thing in the market. Isn't the tongue the organ of sociability, the organ of eloquence, the organ of kindness, the organ of worship?"

The philosopher countered, "Tomorrow I want you to get the worst thing in the market." So once again the servant served four or five courses of tongue. Now Xanthus was truly angry. "Didn't I tell you to get the worst thing in the market?" Again the servant replied, "I did; for isn't the tongue the organ of blasphemy, the organ of defamation, the organ of lying?" The servant had taught the philosopher a great lesson.[35]

---

[35]*The Beam.* Excerpt from "Little But Loud" by Dr. Herschel H. Hobbs, Pastor, First Baptist Church, Oklahoma City, Oklahoma.

The Vice of the Mote Hunter

by J. B. Chapman, D.D.

We speak of mote hunting as a vice, because it does its greatest harm to the hunter himself. It might be a good thing for the neighbor to have help in getting rid of the little particle that has found lodging in his eye; but it would require a helper of clear vision to give such assistance.

The professional mote hunter is not, after all, interested primarily in motes. It is the beam in his own eye that is his concern; and, absurdly, he is not interested in casting out the beam. He is not really righteous enough and strong enough to attack beams, not even in the eyes of other people; so he screams over a mouse to detract attention from the lion.

One of the most familiar manifestations of the mote-hunting vice is *gossip*. The practical effect of gossip is to lower the estimates of listeners as to those who are the subjects of unguarded talk. "Yes, she is good, but ...". "He got the votes, but had you heard ...?" "The work is big, but it is shallow, I believe, in quality." The gossiper does not necessarily consciously lie–he just suggests and intimates. If cornered, he can quickly say, "Oh, I didn't mean that." The gossiper's main authority is "They say," and after this is "I have heard." And yet how many pure women and honest men have been smeared and their influence curtailed by the loose, wagging tongues of thoughtless gossipers!

When the mote hunter attempts to do good, he is likely to select for his crusade some universal evil upon which he can pour his reformatory speech, without taking any chances on being checked up by practical people who demand results; or else he chooses some insignificant subject that contains no vital connection with worthwhile good. He may justify his course by wresting the Scripture about the little foxes that spoil the vines. But the fact still remains that the thing to which he directs his effort is a mote, and not a beam. He gets greatly exercised over some fault in ritual or order in the church, but he gives little time and prayer to a Holy Ghost revival. He sees the faults of the best church members, but he attends no all-night prayer meetings for the reclamation of the straying. He proves his own size by the size of the enemies he selects to fight. Motes, not beams, are his measures.

Minced Oaths

by George H. Seville

A visiting minister was asked to lead in prayer in Sunday school, and when he had finished, a teacher heard one of her girls whisper, "Gosh, what a prayer!" Such an exclamation seems incongruous in expressing one's appreciation of a prayer, but a little thought will lead anyone to the conclusion that "gosh" is not an appropriate word for a Christian on any occasion. When we look into the original meaning of such interjections, we may be surprised that even Christian people are habitual users of expressions which the dictionary terms "minced oaths."

A commonly used interjection is "Gee." It is capitalized in Webster's *New International Dictionary*, and given this definition: "A form of Jesus, used in minced oaths." Two common words and their definitions are these: "Golly: a euphemism for God, used in minced oaths." "Darn, darned, darnation" are said to be "colloquial euphemisms for "damn, damned, damnation." Persons who allow their lips to utter "Goshdarned" quite freely, would be shocked if they realized the real meaning of the word.

Now a professor in a sound seminary, a certain minister was not allowed to use "goodness," "mercy," or "gracious" as exclamations when he was a child. He was inclined to think the restrictions a family peculiarity, merely a parental over-carefulness; but now he can see that it had a sound scriptural basis. The Westminster Shorter Catechism asks, "What is required in the third commandment? The third commandment requireth the holy and reverent use of God's name, titles, *attributes*, ordinances, words and works." Certainly goodness, mercy, graciousness are attributes of God.

The use of minced oaths is quite contrary to the spirit of the New Testament teaching. For example, our Lord Jesus said, "But I say unto you, Swear not at all ... But let your speech be, Yea, yea; Nay, nay; and whatsoever is more than these is of the evil one" (Matthew 5:34, 37 RV). The phrase "whatsoever is more than these" suggests the use of an exclamation or an expletive, which is defined as "something added merely as a filling; especially a word, letter, or syllable not necessary to the sense, but inserted to fill a vacancy."

James, in writing his epistle repeats almost exactly the words of Christ quoted above, but adds the warning: " ... that ye fall not under judgment" (James 5:12). That last word recalls our Lord's declaration, "But I say unto you, that every idle word that men shall speak, they shall give account thereof in the day of judgment. For by thy words thou shalt be justified, and by thy words thou shalt be condemned" (Matthew 12:36-37). If we try to excuse ourselves by saying that these exclamations slips through our lips unawares, we need to heed the Holy Spirit's warning in the epistle of James, "If any man thinketh himself to be religious, while he bridleth not his tongue, but deceiveth his heart, this man's religion is vain" (1:26).

James seems puzzled by the same anomaly that puzzles us, namely, the presence of minced oaths on the lips of Christians. Writing of the tongue as a "restless evil ... full of deadly poison," he said. "Therewith bless we the Lord and Father; and therewith curse we men, who are made after the likeness of God; out of the same mouth cometh forth blessing and cursing. My brethren, these things ought not so to be" (James 3:8-10).

While no attempt has been made to give a complete list of all the words in the vocabulary of near profanity, enough has been said to indicate that present day speech has fallen below that standard which Christ set for His disciples. A careless following of others in the use of these common minced oaths will dull our own spiritual sensitiveness, and will weaken our Christian testimony.

To gain the victory in this matter of full obedience to our Lord Jesus, we need to make the prayer of David our daily petition, "Let the words of my mouth and the meditation of my heart, be acceptable in thy sight, O Lord, my strength and my redeemer" (Psalm 19:14).

–*George H. Seville*

George Washington's View on Profanity

George Washington's Orderly Book of August 3, 1776, included this comment:

"The General is sorry to be informed that the foolish and wicked practice of profane swearing, a vice hitherto little known in the American army, is growing into fashion; he hopes the officers will be examples as well as influence endeavor to check it and that both they and the men will reflect that we can have little hope of the blessing of heaven on our arms if we insult it by our impiety and profanity. Added to this, it is a vice so mean and low, without temptation, that every man of sense and character detests and despises it."

He Who Laughs–Lasts

by Larry Hatfield

The old proverb says: "He laughs best who laughs last." But frequently the last laughter our society hears is the laugh track, produced by wires, solder joints, and transistors. What a poor substitute for old-fashioned, belly-shaking, knee-slapping laughter.

What a delight to be around those wealthy souls who light up a room with their spontaneous laughter. These people frequently have happy attacks, and fortunate are those within hearing range. In a world where harshness and howling seemingly outnumber hilarity and hallelujahs, these have discovered the gift that oils the creaking machinery of life.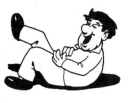

"A merry heart doeth good like a medicine" (Proverbs 17:22). Scientists have studied the effects of laughter on the human body. They have determined the relaxing of tensions and exercise of internal tissue produced by laughter are conducive to better physical health. In other words, "He who laughs–lasts."

How wonderful that God has provided a plethora of things that can overturn a tickle box. Moments unplanned, unrehearsed, totally void of anything artificial are constantly challenging somber expressions. Sour faces and sour dispositions can both be sweetened by a frown turned upside down. What a glorious disorder.

May the laugh tracks gather rust. Who needs them? Have a real good laugh. Enjoy a snicker, chuckle, or giggle. Life is too short to look pickled, polished, and preserved. Besides many a nagging problem has been cured by a good horselaugh. It's often just what the doctor ordered.

Laughter is Universal

Babies start giggling by about 4 months of age, sometimes earlier. Most of us don't need laugh lessons, and we don't need experts to tell us that a good guffaw reduces tension, clears the mind, and lifts the spirits.

But there actually is a branch of medicine–called *gelotology*– that studies the effects of laughing on the human body. Gelotologist William Fry, MD, of Stanford University has been researching health and humor since 1953. In the *Journal of the American Medical Association*, he has reported that laughter can improve cardiovascular fitness by lowering both blood pressure and heart rate after briefly raising them. Breathing patterns are changed, with deeper exhalations and increased ventilation that gets more oxygen into the bloodstream. Laughing reduces pain perception, Fry has found, and also helps break the muscle spasm/pain cycle common in rheumatism. It appears to strengthen the immune system response, and a hearty belly laugh certainly gives your abdominal muscles a workout. If you can't muster up a laugh, try grinning. Several studies have shown that even a faked smile can change your mood for the better![36]

Lighten up—Laugh Your Way to Good Health

by *Nick Gallo*

Most people readily agree that a good laugh makes them feel better. Now, evidence shows that humor's benefits may be more powerful and long-lasting than once believed.

Bubbles and Hope

In Schenectady, New York, patients at the Sunnyview Hospital and Rehabilitation Center hit the road to recovery in part by visiting the "humor room" on the third floor. They can check out funny books, tapes, and music or such mirth-makers as clown noses, balloons, and bottles of bubble soap. A poster on a wall reminds visitors to take a "humor break."

"Humor makes patients happy," says Connelly Bruner-Todt, hospital humor coordinator. "And happy patients usually work harder to recover."

Laughter, say many medical experts, is good for those who are sick–and for those who want to stay well.

William F. Fry, M.D., likens laughter to "inner jogging." Fry, associate professor of clinical psychiatry at Stanford University, has studied the effects of laughter for 30 years. Laughing 100 times a day, he says is the cardiovascular equivalent of 10 minutes of rowing.

---

[36]*Pentecostal Evangel*, August 23, 1992.

The latest research bears out Dr. Fry's findings. A good belly laugh exercises your heart as well as your circulatory and respiratory systems. Laugh out loud and you're likely to get your facial, shoulder, and diaphragm muscles into the act, too.

You can practice humor therapy on your own when friends or relatives are laid up. Your efforts could very well speed their recovery. When Green, University of Michigan Hospitals' "Good Humor Lady," visited a friend with leukemia, she changed the room's "view" with posters of city-scapes, mountains, and oceans. She also brought in a steady stream of cartoon books, balloons, and toys.

Each visit, Green filled a dish with different treats such as chocolate kisses and strawberries. "The hospital staff said they'd never seen anyone react to that kind of chemotherapy as well as my friend did," says Green.

Next time you pay a hospital visit, you might be able to follow Green's example by bringing a humor scrapbook filled with funny cartoons and clips. Or bring colorful posters, mobiles, or a "cheer-board," a bulletin board with humorous sayings and pictures.

Don't force laughter. Go slow and gauge whether the patient is coping with his or her illness before stimulating the funny bone.

Laughter, of course, is only part of the equation for staying well and recovering from illness. But an enduring sense of humor, especially combined with other inner resources such as faith and optimism, appears to be a potent force for better health.

Learn to Laugh

Build for yourself a strong box,
Fashion each part with care;
Fit it with hasp and padlock,
Put all your troubles there.
Hide therein all your failures,
And each bitter cup and quaff;
Lock all your heartaches within it,
Then sit on the lid and laugh.
Tell no one of its contents,
Never its secrets share;
Drop in your cares and worries,
Keep them forever there.
Hide them from sight so completely,
The world will never dream half;
Fasten the top down securely,
Then, sit on the lid and laugh!
–Author unknown

Of course the preceding poem is slanted from a worldly viewpoint but we can apply it in a spiritual sense, i.e., the "strong box" can represent our precious Lord and to Him we bring all our burdens, heartaches, cares and worries. He exchanges them all for His joy and laughter!

Healing Power of Laughter

In the *Seattle Community School News* I read some announcements of the class sessions for April 8 to June 3, 1985. One subject was entitled: *HEALING POWER OF LAUGHTER.* A notation concerning this subject stated:

"Learn to apply the laughter prescription to facilitate physical and emotional healing and well-being. Humor applied to home, workplace and social setting helps you tackle life's toughest problems. Participate in fun-filled exercises which promote positive emotions, reduce pain and prioritize goals. Instructor is health educator and family specialist with training and personal experience in the subject. *Ballard High School, W 7-9 p.m. Date 2-18 to 3-4 = 3 weeks. Fee: $15.*"

Laughter and Fitness

Laughter is called by *Dr. Fry, Jr.* a kind of *"stationary jogging—there is hardly a system in the body a hearty laugh doesn't stimulate."* The actual muscular activity from your lungs and diaphragm in the spasmodic explosion of laughing is nothing less than powerful exercise for chest and abdominal muscles as well as all internal glands and organs! *Start off each morning with a hearty laugh/exercise session.* Here's how:

Stand with feet about 24 inches apart, knees bent slightly, arms bent and overhead, slightly in back of your head. *Now, bring the palms of your hands down and slap them hard on your knees. Next swing your bent arms back overhead and vigorously laugh!*

After a few tries, your laughter will be genuine and so will the degree of exercise it provides. Keep this up for 5 to 10 minutes. Results will amaze you! It energizes your muscles and glands, makes you feel real good all over – and it even chases away the blues! This is powerful medicine to restore health, fitness and good cheer.

A few years ago, Norman Cousins, famous editor of *Saturday Review* actually cured himself of a deadly form of spinal arthritis [ankylosing spondylitis] using massive doses of vitamin C—*and a tremendous amount of laughter every day.* The combination of nutrition and laughter made his body and mind fit, setting the stage for Nature [God] to produce a "cure," when doctors called his condition "helpless." (Norman Cousins cured his condition and published a landmark article detailing this in the *New England Journal of Medicine*, entitled "The Anatomy of an Illness.")

Recently, in a study by Dr. Stanley Tan and Lee Berk at Loma Linda University (California) volunteers watched a comedy video for one hour. Blood samples were taken before, during and after watching the video. The samples showed that there were measurable positive changes in the immune system after the volunteers watched the video. From the above examples, one must conclude that laughter, joy and happiness should be your natural state–not something you must earn. *More than 60 years ago, the world famous Physical Culturist, Bernarr Macfadden wrote about laughter as a form of exercise.* He and his followers derived so much benefit from laughter as an exercise that he called it his "Laugh Cure." You will, too, once you try it!

–Author Unknown

Feel Funny, Feel Good

Like exercise, laughter reduces stress. Once laughter stops, blood pressure drops below normal for a brief period. Breathing slows down. Muscular tension subsides. The result: Most people feel a relaxed afterglow.

Regular "doses" of laughter may even have dramatic effects in combating disease. Several years ago, Norman Cousins, former editor of *The Saturday Review*, reported in his best-selling book, *Anatomy of an Illness*, that laughter helped him recover from a progressive, connective-tissue disease. Instead of languishing in a hospital bed, Cousins began watching Marx brothers' movies and reruns of *Candid Camera*, and taking massive doses of vitamin C. He discovered that 10 minutes of genuine belly laughter brought him two hours of pain-free sleep. Medical tests confirmed that his physical condition improved after laughing.

Few doctors advise anyone to "laugh off" a serious illness or to expect belly-jiggling chortles to be a medical cure-all. But many believe that "humor therapy" has serious benefits.

Take Two Chuckles

Texas Tech University held an experiment involving students' tolerance for pain and noted that this increased following the viewing of a comedy tape.

Biochemically, laughter seems to cause the release of natural pain-killers that combat arthritis and other inflammatory conditions. It may also slow the release of some stress hormones.

"When all the evidence is in, I believe we'll find that laughter is a total body experience," believes Dr. Fry. "All the major systems participate."

Laughter also appears to be one of the best antidepressants available. Like a ray of sunshine, it softens emotional pain, brightens outlook, and broadens perspective.

Laughter is No Joke

Hospitals and nursing homes are starting to treat laughter seriously: At Duke University Hospital in Durham, North Carolina, oncology recreation therapists offer a "laugh-mobile" cart stocked with funny books, games, and monologues by such humorists as Bill Cosby and Erma Bombeck. Lila Green, a consultant, conducts workshops for health-care workers to reduce stress and prevent burn-out at The University of Michigan Hospitals in Ann Arbor. Mental-health therapists, too, see the value of humor in maintaining health. Laughter helps release pent-up emotions and purge painful feelings, notes Waleed Salameh, Ph.D., a San Diego clinical psychologist.

Section 4
Related Items on Health

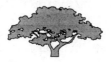

The Elderly

Setting the Record Straight

Tales of the deterioration of the aging brain are just that–*tales*. For example:

Vast numbers of brain cells *do not* begin to disappear annually once you reach voting age. To the contrary, says Marian Diamond, Ph.D., neuroanatomist at the University of California in Berkeley, the greatest loss of brain cells occurs very early in life, not later.

Whether you are 35 or 85, you no more need to look forward to senility than you do to heart disease or lung cancer. The healthy brain of an active adult is one of the most resilient organs Mother Nature [God] has given us.

The overall thinking skills of a 55-year-old are almost always markedly superior to those of a 25-year-old. Studies by K. Warner Schaie, Ph.D., professor of human development at Pennsylvania State University, show that a challenged brain simply never quits learning.

Go Ahead, Cry Your Eyes Out

Laughter may be the best medicine, but there's a great case for crying out loud. "Having a good cry relieves stress and makes you feel better," says Dr. William Frey, who serves as the director of psychiatry research at the Ramsey Clinic in St. Paul, Minnesota. Studies show that people with stress-related disorders like ulcers and colitis cry less than healthy people, Frey adds.

And experts believe that high blood pressure, arthritis and tension headaches can become more severe when a patient's emotions are suppressed. We cry for many reasons–happy and sad, says Frey, author of Crying: The Mystery of Tears (Winston Press). "It's a rare person who never sheds tears of sorrow, joy, anguish or ecstasy," he explains. "Even those who seldom are known to cry for personal reasons may be brought to tears watching a sad movie or play."

But there are times when it's best not to shed tears. For example, women who shed tears at the office are often seen as weak and manipulative by their co-workers.

Confidential to hurting in Hilton Head, S.C.: Give your grief a chance to express itself. Cry your eyes out. Let yourself go and let the tears flow. It's healthy. Don't try to put on a "brave" show. It takes honesty, courage, strength and real manliness for a man to express his emotions. The weak man hides.
–From the *"Dear Abby"* Column in *L.A. Examiner*

Hugging is Healthy

Written by Mrs. Elliott

Hugging is healthy: It helps the body's immunity system, it keeps you healthier, it cures depression, it reduces stress, it induces sleep, it's invigorating, it's rejuvenating, it has no unpleasant side effects, and hugging is nothing less than a miracle drug.

Hugging is all natural: It is organic, naturally sweet, no pesticides, no preservatives, no artificial ingredients and 100 percent wholesome.

Hugging is practically perfect: There are no movable parts, no batteries to wear out, no periodic checkups, low energy consumption, high energy yield, inflation-proof, nonfattening, no monthly payments, no insurance requirements, theft-proof, nontaxable, non-polluting and, of course, fully returnable.

The following analysis of a person weighing 140 lbs. is given by Dr. E. F. Lawson of London: Enough water to fill a 10-gallon keg, enough fat for seven bars of soap, enough carbon for 9,000 lead pencils, enough phosphorus to make 2,200 match heads, sufficient magnesium for one dose of salts, enough iron to make a medium-sized nail, sufficient lime to whitewash a chicken coop, and enough sulphur to rid a terrier dog of fleas!

The Brain

There are 120 trillion brain connections in the head. Capillaries in the body, which, if laid end to end, would wrap five times around the earth, are in such synchronized working order that they carry blood, nutrition, and oxygen to the entire body.

The Brain is a pinkish-gray mushy membrane slightly larger than a grapefruit, weighs less than 3 pounds, yet a computer capable of handling a single brain's output would cover the entire earth. The brain sorts one hundred million bits of data from the eyes, ears, nose and other sensory outposts each second, yet uses far less electricity than an average light bulb. The brain itself feels no pain, yet controls pain and directs the grand orchestra that includes all our senses and bodily functions, our emotions and the sense of our place in the universe.

The brain consists of a lump of "gray matter" whose various segments control everything from our ability to walk and talk to the fear, or joy, we experience when flying.

The human brain is a wonderful thing. It starts working the moment you are born, and never stops until you stand up to speak in public! *George Jessel* (Jewish entertainer).

Mental Malady

Motor Mouth

by Nikki Bridges and Kevin Mahady

We all have experienced problem talkers, the conversation killers who selfishly yak on and on.

Well, it may be a mental malady, out of their control. Experts now are starting to recognize incessant talking as a psychological problem.

Psychotherapist Stephen Bank says incessant talking can cause problems with relationships, work productivity and even profit.

He says it's not because Chatty Kathys are conversationally selfish–it's just that they haven't learned the mechanics of conversation. That is why they run roughshod over other folks' comments instead of learning to be quiet and listen.

He says insecurity sets people talking, too, because they think quantity makes up for a lack of conversational quality.

If you think you are an insufferable speaker, Bank says watch for vague, restless looks from bored listeners. Or ask your best friend, who is likely to be truthful, about your level of talking.

Strange Fears of the Mind

There is an old Arabian proverb that tells about Pestilence, riding to place a scourge upon a camp. When asked how many of the encampment he would take, Pestilence replied, "Only one-third of the people do I take with me." And he rode on.

Some time later he was seen again and accosted by the tribe who accused him: "You said you would take only one-third of our people with you, yet over one-half of the whole tribe is gone."

"I kept my word," replied Pestilence. "I took only those that I said I would–*Fear* took all the rest."

Fear is called *phobia* and is opposite to faith. Following is an excerpt from an article by Dr. J. G. Molner (with some changes I have made) in answer to a teen-ager who had a problem of fainting. He began by explaining the fear of closed-in places (*claustophobia*), then listed different phobias.

How phobias develop is not easy to explain. Some people are afraid of open spaces, of water, of germs, of all sorts of things. There are more than 250 identified phobias. As examples, some people are afraid of choking. *Theophobia* is being afraid of God, if you can conceive of such a thing. But it occurs. There's a condition called *hydro-phobophobia*, meaning a fear of hydrophobia, and *ballistophobia*, which is fear of missiles. There are phobias involving snakes, sleep, colors, fire, heights, ideas, crowds, thunder, trains, bees, dogs, devils, odors.

There is even *auroraphobia*, meaning fear of the northern lights, and *phobophobia* that is fear of one's own fears. ... There is *hygrophobia*, which means a fear of moisture, but I can not find a term for small boys who are afraid of taking baths–maybe that isn't a phobia. Maybe they just don't like 'em.

I don't belittle phobias. We may be astonished, or amused at some of them, but they are real, and few are common, like fear of lightning, and some are uncommon, like *levophobia*, a fear of things on one's left side! ... *Claustrophobia* is a morbid fear of enclosed places. It is uncommon with teen-agers, but it can occur at any age.

My Added Notes

Hypochrondria is a mental disorder which is accompanied by melancholy and depression and is often caused by *self-pity* and *self-centeredness.* Following are types of Phobias (alphabetically listed):

Acaraphobia–Fear of itching
Acrophobia–Fear of high places
Agoraphobia–Fear of crossing or being large, open spaces
Aichmophobia–Fear of sharp instruments
Ailurophobia–Fear of cats
Algophobia–Fear of pain
Androphobia–Morbid dislike of the male sex
Anthrophobia–Morbid dread of human society
Autophobia–Fear of self
Batophobia–Fear of passing near or among high objects
Biennophobia–Fear of slime
Brontophobia–Fear of thunderstorms
Cherophobia–Fear of gaiety
Cibophobia–Abnormal loathing of food
Claustrophobia–Fear of being in closed or narrow spaces
Cremnophobia–Fear of precipices
Cynophobia–Fear of dogs
Dorapobia–Morbid dread of the skin or fur of animals
Dromophobia–Fear of running
Eratophobia–Morbid dislike for sexual love
Ergasiophobia–Morbid aversion to work; also, undue fear of performing surgical operations
Erythrophobia–Fear of blushing

Gamophobia–Morbid fear of marriage
Gephydrophobia–Fear of crossing bridges
Graphophobia–Fear of writing
Gynephobia–Morbid aversion to women
Hydrophobia–Fear of water
Kakorrephiaphobia–Fear of failure
Maleusiophobia–Fear of pregnancy
Microphobia–Fear of germs
Monophobia–Fear of being alone
Mysophobia–Fear of dirt
Mythophobia–Fear of making false statements
Necrophobia–Fear of death
Neophobia–Fear of new things
Nosemaphobia–Fear of illness
Nyctophobia–Fear of the dark
Oclophobia–Fear of crowds
Pediophobia–Fear of children
Phgonophobia–Fear of beards
Phobophobia–Fear of fear
Photophobia–Fear of light
Pnigophobia–Fear of choking
Triakaidekaphobia–Fear of seating 13 at a table
Sitophobia–Morbid fear of eating
Zoophobia–fear of animals

Remedy to Eliminate Phobias

A perfect remedy to eliminate fear (phobia) is found in the following verses of the Bible:

*"And thou shalt **love** the LORD thy God with all thine heart, and with all thy soul, and with all thy might"* (Deuteronomy 6:5). This means that the spirit (heart), soul, and body (might) of man is to love the Lord.

*" There is **no fear in love**; but **perfect love** CASTETH OUT FEAR: because fear hath torment. **He that feareth is not made perfect in love**"* (1 John 4:18).

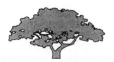

The Cook or the Book, Which?

Cook Stove Apostasy

The Cooking Squad vs. The Praying Band

The early church *prayed* in the **Upper Room**; the Twentieth Century church *cooks* in the **supper room**.

Today the **supper room** has taken the place of the **Upper Room**! *Play* has taken the place of *prayer*, and *feasting* the place of *fasting*. There are more *full stomachs* in the church than there are **bended knees** and **broken hearts**. There is more fire in the **kitchen range** than there is in the *church pulpit*. When you build a fire in the church kitchen it often, if not altogether, puts out the fire in the **church pulpit**; *ice cream* chills the fervor of *spiritual life*.

The early Christians were not *cooking* in the **supper room** the day when the **Holy Ghost** came but they were *praying* in the **Upper Room**! They were not *waiting* on *tables*, they were *waiting* on *God*. They were not *waiting* for the fire from the *stove*, but for the *fire* from *above*.

They were *detained* by the *command of God*, and not *entertained* by the *cunning* of *men*. They were all *filled* with the *Holy Ghost*, *NOT* stuffed with *stew* or *roast*.

Oh! I would like to see the *cooking squad* put out, and the *praying band* put in. Less *ham* and *sham* and more *heaven*, less *pie* and more *piety*. Less *cook*, and more use for the old, *old Book*. Put out the fire in the church kitchen and build it on the *church altar*.

More *love* and more *life*. Fewer *dinners* and get after *sinners*. Let us have a church full of *waiters*, *waiting* on *God*, a church full of *servers*, serving *God* and waiting for His dear *Son* from *heaven*.

—*Selected*

Heavenly Menu

Have you ever partaken of the *Heavenly Menu* in God's Word? This Menu includes:

"**Honey** out of the rock" (Psalm 81:16), the sweetness of grace in Christ.

"Finest of the **wheat**," (margin: "fat of wheat,"(Psalm 81:16), the spiritual vitamins of God's promises.

"True **bread** from heaven," (John 6:32). Jesus is the embodiment of those truths which are the life of the Spirit.

"**Corn** of heaven" (Psalm 78:24-25), a name for **manna**, a corn not produced of earth, sustenance from above, *angels' food.*

"Strong **meat** of the Word" (Hebrews 5:14), the deeper things of revelation for the mature servant.

"Twelve manner of *fruits*" (Revelation 22:2), a variety of seasonable desserts to delight the taste of the saint.

"**Wine and Milk**" (Isaiah 55:1), wine, symbol of the joy of divine wisdom, Proverbs 9:5-6 and milk, symbol of the rudimentary Gospel truths, 1 Peter 2:2.

"**Water** clear as crystal" (Revelation 22:1), refreshing from the river of God's pleasures. Psalm 36:8).[37]

Eating to the Glory of God

by Abbie C. Morrow Brown

"Whether therefore ye eat, or drink, or whatsoever ye do, do all to the glory of God" (1 Corinthians 10:31).

Suffering and "glory" are inseparable. "Even the death of the cross" must precede "wherefore God hath highly exalted" (Philippians 2:5-12). Suffering is absolutely essential to the obtaining of any glory. Luke 17:24-25; 24:26; Romans 8:17-18; Hebrews 2:9; 1 Peter 1:7; 4:12-14.

We suffer for Christ when we crucify ourselves. We suffer with Christ when others crucify us. We suffer for love of Christ when we crucify our "earthly nature with its passions and its cravings," Galatians 5:24; when we through the Spirit "put an end to the evil habits of the body" (Romans 8:13, Twentieth Century Version).

---

[37]*Prophecy Monthly*, January 1959, p.47.

Eating too much; eating too fast; eating too often; eating too rich food; eating too many things at one meal; eating and murmuring, or complaining, or fault finding; eating and talking about foods instead of the things of the Kingdom; eating and gossiping instead of communing; all these are "evil habits" that it costs much to absolutely put to death.

You eat to the glory of God when you eat enough, and no more; eat very slowly, chewing each mouthful of food until it becomes liquid; eat wholesome food; eat, thankful for anything; eat joyfully, though the food be ill-cooked and badly served; eat patiently, though there be delay in the service; eat in liberty but "do not make your freedom an opportunity of self-indulgence" (Galatians 5:13); eat in love, with no desire for anything different or anything cooked differently, because what is before you is your heavenly Father's provision for you. Eat in due season for strength and not for pleasure (Mark 16:18; Ecclesiastes 10:17).

A long stride toward crucifying the flesh is taken when one habitually goes without breakfast. This has often proved true even among worldlings who only abstained on purely physical grounds.

Truly, "the children of this world are in their generation wiser than the children of light" (Luke 16:8). Through the simple giving up of the morning meal, drunkards have been reformed, tobacco users have abandoned the weed, coffee inebriates have laid aside this stimulant, gluttons have become moderate eaters, and the lustful have overcome evil desires.

Of all the choice blessings the heavenly Father has bestowed upon me through the years I count the grace of going without breakfast the greatest.

From the time I prayed for the Lord to help me to go without breakfast, all desire for food in the early morning left me. The breakfast hour is now devoted to prayerful reading of the Bible for personal profit.

Going without breakfast was not a hard and fast rule of bondage. It was a great delight, which I was only willing to forego if we were visiting and friends were distressed and asked me to eat.

Omitting the early morning meal has many advantages. It gives one time to be absolutely alone with God. It makes possible the habit of family prayer. It tends to build one up spiritually. It quickens all the mental faculties. It wonderfully conduces to physical health. It takes away dyspepsia and kindred stomach troubles. It does away with almost one-third of the cooking and dishwashing. It saves money which could be devoted to the Lord's work.

Two meals a day is surely God's best for man, for it is written, "Woe to thee, O land, when thy king is a child and thy princes eat *in the morning*! Blessed art thou, O land, when thy king is the son of nobles, and thy princes *eat in due season* for strength, and not for drunkenness" (Ecclesiastes 10:16-17).

The children of Israel in the wilderness did not have an early meal, for they had to wait until the dew was gone up from the ground before they gathered the tiny seed. Then it was dried thoroughly, ground into flour and baked or boiled (Exodus 16:14-23).

The word *breakfast* is not in the Bible, either in the Hebrew or the Greek. On the seashore, when Jesus said, "Come and *dine*," He used a Greek word meaning the principal meal of the day.

In Luke 14:12 when referring to the meals of the day, Jesus said: "When thou makest a *dinner* or a *supper* ..."

I know of no thought of God for the overcoming people of God that the adversary fights more persistently than *fasting* from breakfast or *fasting generally.*

"Whether therefore ye eat, or drink, or whatsoever ye do, do all to the glory of God" (1 Corinthians 10:31).

Some "Funnies" About Diet

Charlotte Spitzer is on a slow fat diet.
Don't you mean *low* fat?
No, *slow* fat! She eats whatever she wants and slowly gets fatter!

Dieting

The fashion, now, is to reduce,
To keep the girlish look;
You must not eat a single thing
Not in the diet book.
The calories must be kept down;
It's really quite a trick
To eat enough to keep alive,
Keep slim and looking chic.
But when the pains of hunger grow,
The suffering is great,
For those who've been a little stout,
To make that hunger wait.

The Overthrow of King Gastric Juicibus

There was a mighty monarch called King Gastric Juicibus. He ruled over a kingdom called Stomachiticus. And the only way to his kingdom was through a long, long, lane called Aesophagus.

One day when King Gastric Juicibus sat on his throne enjoying peace and plenty, he looked down that long, long lane and beheld approaching one of his bitter enemies–Lobster Saladibus.

King Gastric Juicibus arose quickly from his throne, girded on his armor, strapped on his sword, and prepared himself to do battle.

They fought for hours and hours. Finally King Gastric Juicibus was victorious, and he overcame Lobster Saladibus and tied him up in a knot and threw him over into one corner of his kingdom.

But hardly had he sat down again on his throne when, looking down that long, long lane, he beheld another enemy approaching. This time it was his deadly enemy, Chicken-a-la-Kingibus.

He arose again from his throne and buckled on his armor and strapped on his sword. They fought for hours and hours and hours, and finally when the strength of King Gastric Juicibus was almost exhausted, he prevailed and overthrew his enemy, Chicken-a-la-Kingibus, and tied him up in a knot and threw him over into another corner of his kingdom.

But King Gastric Juicibus had hardly sat down again on his throne till, looking again down that long, long lane, he beheld approaching his most deadly enemy, Mince Pie a-la-Modibus.

King Gastric Juicibus again buckled on his armor and strapped on his sword and prepared himself to do battle. They fought for hours and hours and hours and hours. But this time King Gastric Juicibus was not the victor. He was overthrown by Mince Pie a-la-Modibus. And Mince Pie a-la-Modibus tied up King Gastric Juicibus into a knot and threw him over into a corner of his kingdom.

Then Mince Pie a-la-Modibus went over to Chicken a-la-Kingibus and untied him and set him on his feet. Then he went over to Lobster Saladibus and untied him and set him on his feet. Then Mince Pie a-la-Modibus said to Chicken a-la-Kingibus and Lobster Saladibus, "Come on, boys, let's go upstairs!"

A Hostess' Lament

I've cooked a roast
And mashed potatoes,
Baked two pies
And sliced tomatoes,
Polished silver
And set the table.
I only hope that
I am able
To be charming
And keep quiet
If someone says,
"I'm on a diet."

–*Mrs. Olson*

A Way to Slim Down

An infallible way to slim down: Live on the sixth floor. When a meal is served, take one bite, then fling the fork out of the window. Walk downstairs, retrieve the fork, and climb back up. Repeat until your plate is empty!

Eating Habits

Winston Churchill used to worry his doctors because of his eating habits, that sometimes he would eat only one meal a day; other times, five or six. According to Carlton Fredericks, a nutritionist, Sir Winston followed this line of thinking: "Don't eat by clocktime. Eat by bellytime."

Epitaph on a Tombstone

Here doth lieth
Walter Pryet
Reason whyeth
Fast-food diet.

Poundage Paradox?

Ruth M. Walsh, San Jose, California

Women's magazines
Are really riots:
50 pages of mouth-watering recipes,
50 pages of reducing diets!

Only Fit

My clothing, bursting when I try it,
Has forced me to begin a diet,
Which I find terrible and hard,
Which leaves my temper battle-scarred,
But with which somehow I can cope
As long as I am spurred by hope
That soon, in just a few weeks hence,
I'll have a fitting recompence.

Kept Weighting

Erma Bombeck

Me go on a diet? It's no use! I know that now. All those years when my knees rubbing together whispered "NO, no," but there was a "Yes, yes" in my mouth, I fought the battle.

All those years when I lost 10 pounds every Monday (five in my neck and five in my bust), I hung in there.

All those years when I embraced cottage cheese as a formal religion, I gave it my all.

But after yesterday, I have to admit I'm beaten. I'm fighting the battle alone.

It started in the morning when I faced the refrigerator with my hand over my heart and once again pledged allegiance to hunger. I poured myself a half glass of tomato juice mixed with half a glass of buttermilk and tossed it down. I felt virtuous.

At lunch, I threw down a cup of bouillon and pretended celery was wicked.

I had dinner ready to serve by 3:30 in the afternoon. It was well-balanced and would be totally satisfying. Broiled fish, an oil-free salad, asparagus and an apple.

At 4:00 p.m. I looked at the dinner again. It looked pale, so I surrounded it with a fruit salad with coconut in it.

At 4:30, with nothing to do, I rolled out a pan of biscuits to pop into the oven.

By 5:00, the asparagus looked naked without a sauce, so I opted for a Hollandaise.

By 5:30, I was furious. How dare my husband be late and force me to obesity? I added whipped potatoes to the meal.

By 5:45, as I stood watching the driveway, I got a horrifying feeling. How could you possibly serve dry whipped potatoes? I added a pan of gravy.

By 6:00, the fish looked terminal. I decided to get my husband's mind off the small main course by giving him a robust appetizer. I rolled out those little butter, cheese and flour things stuffed with olives and popped them in the oven.

By 6:15, I sliced the apples and covered them with a pie. At 6:30, my husband walked into the kitchen. "I'm home," he shouted brightly.

"You animal! You don't care about other people at all. How they look. How they feel about themselves. If I go to my grave with pantyhose around my hips, let it be on your conscience." He pretended he didn't know what I was talking about.

An Overactive Fork

A friend of an obese person asked a doctor about his weight problem, and after an examination the doctor announced: "I found your problem: You're suffering from an over-active fork."

A Rule for Food

Dine with little, sup with less; do better still: sleep supperless.
—*Ben Franklin*

Tough Part of Diet

The toughest part of a diet isn't watching what you eat. It's watching what everyone else eats!

Calorie Counter's Prayer

(Apologies to Shepherd/King David who wrote the 23rd Psalm.)

The Lord is my shepherd, I shall not want,
He maketh me lie down and do push-ups.
He restoreth my waistline.
He leadeth me past the refrigerator
for my own sake,

He maketh me to partake of the green beans
instead of the potatoes.
He leadeth me past the pizzeria.
Yea, though I walk through the bakery,
I shall not falter, for thou art with me;
Thy Tab and Fresca, they comfort me.
Thou preparest a diet for me
in the presence of my enemies.
Thou anointest my lettuce
with low-cal oil.
My cup will not overflow.
Surely Ry-Krisp and D-Zerta shall follow me
all the days of my life,
And I will live with pains
of hunger forever, Amen.

A Planned Garden

Okay, Uncle Cosmo ... This year we're gonna *plan* our garden. Now let's figure out what vegetables we really like to eat ... Let's go over our eating habits meal by meal. Breakfast?

Yea ... put in a row of glazed donuts!

Section 6
Fasting

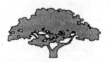

Following are excerpts from the article entitled:

Is Fasting for Today?

by Douglas Batchelder

In a fast-food world, fasting seems a bit silly, an antique of the Old Testament, something fitting for a prophet in Israel but hardly practical for a believer soon to enter the 21st century.

Many regard fasting as a childish ploy designed to twist the arm of the Almighty, assuming it's something a sophisticated Christian would never undertake.

Others consider fasting a quick cure for spiritual ailments—a sure way to recapture the fire and fervor of the first-century church. They make it a means of gaining apostolic excitement. They use it to spice up an otherwise tasteless Christian experience—as if, by denying food to the body, they can make up for the malnourishment of their soul.

Then there are others who honestly admit, "I'm confused." The thought of fasting fascinates them, but they neglect it. Like an old, valuable tool, it's tucked away in storage because they have no idea how to use it.

Who is right? The answer requires tackling several basic questions.

What is Fasting?

In the Bible, four words denote fasting. *Nesteia* means "to not eat"; *asitos* means "without grain or food." These two Greek words reinforce our common understanding of fasting—going without food.

The Hebrew words are more expansive. *Tsum*, the root word for fast, means "to cover the mouth"; *anah* means "to afflict or humble oneself." These words imply that there is a purpose to this practice of abstaining from eating.

Essentially, fasting is voluntarily denying the body something for a specific purpose. It relates to the practice of one's faith. Although not eating is the most common type of fast, the object denied is not always food.

In 2 Samuel 12:16, David denies himself sleep during his fast, as does King Darius in Daniel 6:18. The king also denies himself the pleasures of entertainment as he fasts for Daniel's well-being while Daniel is in the den of lions. Paul refers to a fast that calls for abstaining from sexual relations for a brief period of time for the purpose of prayer (1 Corinthians 7:5).

Fasts can be categorized in this way: *Formal*—those occurring on the day of atonement and practiced together by all Israel in obedience to Leviticus 16:29, which required that the nation as individuals humble themselves.

Informal—the spontaneous response to a situation beyond one's control. For example, David's fast for his dying infant son reveals the warrior's soul as dependent upon God. Helpless and humble, he spontaneously fasted. Such fasts touch the heart of God.

Ritual—those practiced by the Pharisees and purposely avoided by the Lord Jesus. Instituted to commemorate special events, these fasts became an exercise of egotism, designed to impress others.

Christ had little use for the ritual fast or the self-righteous who practiced it (Matthew 6:16-18; 9:13-17). It existed to prove that a man could be [seemingly] righteous without being right with God.

How Does Scripture Treat Fasting?

Scripture presents at least three distinct reasons for fasting. The first is to express sorrow. David mourned his closest friend's death (2 Samuel 1:11-12). Nehemiah fasted in sorrow over the reproach and condition of Jerusalem (Nehemiah 1:4).

This type of fasting seems normal; many people refuse to eat when they're upset. But to find a man fasting in sorrow over his nation's sin (Daniel 9) is unusual. It's the response of a soul touched by God's holiness and aware of how far short he has fallen.

People then, like people today, felt no sorrow for sin because so few appreciated the holiness of God. But Daniel did. Perhaps that's why he's called "highly esteemed" by God.

Closely related to fasting as an expression of sorrow is fasting as a sign of repentance. In Joel 2:12, God tells the people of Israel to return to Him and to demonstrate the sincerity of their repentance by weeping, mourning and fasting.

As a sign of repentance, fasting takes a slightly different twist in Jonah 3 and 1 Kings 21. Nineveh and King Ahab fast in repentance to avert God's judgment, and the judgment was averted—not because they fasted, but because they repented.

God is interested in the heart, not in perfunctory actions of any sort, whether fasting, giving, worship or service. Insincere spiritual incantations cannot fool the Lord.

The third reason for fasting, and the most expansive, is to make a request of God.

Knowing that a pagan culture watched him, Ezra fasted to request safe passage on his journey to Jerusalem. Esther, too, requested protection and deliverance when she fasted before going in to King Ahasuerus, who had recently banished another queen for stepping out of line.

Other requests made of God through prayer and fasting include: prayer for victory in battle (Jehoshaphat, 2 Chronicles 20); prayer for healing (David, 2 Samuel 12); prayer for deliverance from satanic power (Jesus, disciples, Matthew 4:17); and prayer regarding afflictions and great needs—a general category that could include just about any serious situation (David, Psalm 109).

One of the most significant reasons for fasting occurs in Acts 13 and 14. The early church leaders, and perhaps entire congregations, fasted and prayed before choosing missionaries and elders.

Perhaps churches and mission fields would be spared many problems if local churches would be prayer and fasting screen out unqualified people. No decision-making issues are more pressing; serious thought and prayer is a must. If the choices were less casual, we'd have fewer casualties.[38]

Fasting for Health and Healing [39]

"Beloved, I wish above all things that thou mayest prosper and be in health, ..." (3 John 2).

"... thine health shall spring forth speedily: ..." (Isaiah 58:8).

God has no vested interests in sickness and infirmity. We may say that it is His general desire, as it was the apostle's for his friend Gaius, that His people should be in health. Exceptions to this do not negative the general rule. If this were not the case He would never have equipped the human body with its own wonderful healing powers or His Church with a healing ministry.

Included in the many blessed results of God's chosen fast is the promise. 'Your healing shall spring up speedily.' Is this a natural healing made possible by the fast, or a supernatural healing? We believe the promise embraces both possibilities.

Fasting, as we have already stressed, has a way of detaching us from the world of the material, so that our thinking becomes rightly orientated, focused on God and the unseen world of which He is the center. This inevitably results in a release of faith, which is 'the assurance of things hoped for, the conviction of things not seen' (Hebrews 11:1).

Scripture has recorded some of the mighty things God has wrought down the years for ordinary men and women who dared to believe Him. They have conquered kingdoms, received promises, shut the mouths of lions, quenched raging fire, and even witnessed the resurrection of the dead (Hebrews 11:33-35). It is not therefore surprising

---

[38]Moody Monthly, April, 1983, pp. 36-37.
[39]Excerpt from *God's Chosen Fast* by Arthur Wallis, pp. 80-81.

that, through the quickening of faith which fasting brings, God has often supernaturally fulfilled this promise of healing.

But there is also the natural healing and rejuvenation of the body through fasting, ... Here is a natural boon in which all who fast for any reasonable length may partake. ... From an article in *Christianity Today* we have the following quotation from James Morrison: 'There are multitudes of diseases which have their origin in fullness, and might have their end in fasting.' Without a doubt there are ills that could be cured, or better still prevented, and a better state of general health enjoyed, if fasting coupled with reformed eating habits were practiced. Oblivious of this, man still continues to dig his grave with his knife and fork! ...

Food for Thought

by Reverend Dale Turner, Columnist for *The Seattle Times*

The strongest drive in the body is the drive for food and drink. God has made food delicious, given it a delightful and enticing aroma, and given us an appetite! The Creator evidently intended that eating be one of life's most pleasurable experiences. Unfortunately, it is such a pleasurable experience that we are tempted to eat more than we need.

The proliferation of weight loss programs and diet prescriptions reveals the magnitude of our excesses. As Johnny Carson says, "Obesity is widespread." We can understand why the two questions most often asked in America today are "Where can I park?" and "How can I lose weight?"

Eating and drinking to excess are sources of many of our diseases and infirmities. As a lamp is choked by too much oil and a fire is extinguished by too much wood, so the natural health of the body is destroyed by too much food. Was it the destructive effect of eating or drinking to excess that caused the church fathers to list gluttony among the Seven Deadly Sins? Or is it deeper than that?

The peculiar thing about gluttony is that although its physical penalties may be the heaviest of all the deadly sins, it is the sin that often seems to leave many with the lightest deposit of guilt. I don't remember anyone who feared they weighed too much to be admitted into heaven–or that fatness was a deterrent to salvation.

But it is true that disagreements among religions, denominations and sects have been based more often on the "sinful" qualities of various kinds of foods, rather than upon amounts. Any amount of certain foods, drinks or drugs is believed to be a sin.

There are many erroneous accusations related to obesity. Often those who carry extra pounds are assumed to be gluttonous and are victims of unwarranted prejudice. Such judgments are not only unfair, but unkind. There are many complex factors beyond genuine hunger that contribute to obesity. Worry, loneliness or boredom may encourage us to eat more than we need.

Obesity is not necessarily the result of willful decisions on the part of those who are overweight. Those who are well-informed on the subject of nutrition have convinced me that many obese people have little control over their insatiable desire to eat.

A predisposition to obesity can also come from genetics or an imbalance of body chemistry. I am a late-onset diabetic, and for the past nine years I have had to zig and zag to avoid sugars. Like many of you, I've loved sweets ever since I can remember, so if it were not for diabetes, I could well have had the problem of the portly preacher pictured in a New Yorker cartoon. The minister is being examined by his doctor, who says, "Your body is a temple, and your congregation is too large."

Through the years, I have gleaned countless comments and items from books, newspapers and refrigerator doors, designed to encourage sensitivity to the dangers of excess. Many have been humorous and are helpful because their humor is a handle which helps me remember. But gluttony is really not funny despite all the humorous remarks which have been made about it. "Gluttony is a sin." Let's think about it.

We'd all be better off
If we followed this one rule
Take more food for thought
Take less food for fuel.

In a well-ordered life, reason directs and appetite obeys. There are counselors who will help us if we will listen. When I was young, Jack Dempsey was one of my sports heroes. I was impressed when I heard him say, "Always arise from a meal table feeling that you could eat a little more." That was wise counsel. I have not always followed it, but when I have overeaten, I always regret it.

A word closely related to gluttony which we hear a lot of these days is addiction. From pleasure and choice, from habit or custom, or from addiction, a person may use food, drink or drugs to harmful excess.

In his book "Whatever Became of Sin?" Dr. Karl Menninger says, "Self-administered food, drink and drugs can temporarily affect the way the world is perceived, and it can affect the way we feel about it. ... Gluttony in all its forms is sinful, in that it represents a degree of self-love which is self-destructive, a kind of escapist effort to abandon the prison of self." Reinhold Niebuhr says gluttons abandon the self "by seeking a god in a process or a prison outside the self–or in a subconscious existence." And God says, "Thou shalt have no other gods before me."

Gluttony

The ancient Romans, cannily figuring that an emptied stomach would leave room for repeating the banquet course, built into some of their palaces an extraordinary chamber whose purpose was suggested by its name: *vomitarium*. (The modern reverse twist to this beguiling concept is the use of cathartic salts to drive water and undigested food from the body and thus to prevent it from staying on the person as fat. This is a health-wrecking disruption of body mechanics.)

Over-eating is classified in the same category as drunkenness in the Bible. For example, Proverbs 23:21 declares, *"For the drunkard and the glutton shall come to poverty ..."*.

Dr. Lewis G. Moench, a psychiatrist who addressed the Western Hospital Association at a meeting in Salt Lake City, Utah, stated that some people go on eating binges in the same way others go on alcoholic sprees.

As the old serpent laid low our first parents through *gluttony*, so his weapons are easily turned aside through soberness. We ought to take food in the same way as some take medicine, with such moderation that it may help us to serve God; and with such gratitude, that at each single morsel praise may redound to our Creator.

It's Such a Small Sin, Lord

by Richard L. Harrison

I awoke about 3 a.m. with a burning sensation in the pit of my stomach. This was the second time in one week it had happened. Too many snacks and good times at the table on vacation with friends and family–a simple case of indigestion. I had dismissed it before, but this time the "heartburn" went to the soul, not the body, and I recognized it clearly for what it was–sin.

My wife and I had been reading the Bible daily and had finished the historical books. Again and again we'd read about Israel and Judah's desecration of the temple through idolatry and a host of other repeat offenses against God, which would often be followed by His judgment. I had commented, "How foolish can a people be? Had I been in their place I'd learn to stop desecrating God's temple!"

But I have a temple! Scripture says my body is a temple of the Holy Spirit (1 Corinthians 6:19). More and more I put His "temple" in disrepair. But not out of ignorance. I know what is right and proper to maintain it. Instead, I feed my body high cholesterol; fat, juicy, sodium-filled food; making an occasional, feeble attempt at better choices and stopping when I'm full but not sated.

By abusing the wonderful temple God gave me, I was in active, willful rebellion against His plan for my life. Of course, I rationalized my excesses with a string of excuses: "I worked hard today," "I deserve it," "It's the only food available," "This once won't hurt," "I'll do better tomorrow," "I'm on vacation," "I'll start after the holiday," "I'll offend my hostess if I don't eat it all," "I'll exercise more."

The basic sin is *disobedience*: placing anything–including food–above God's will. The issue is also one of stewardship. *How am I treating God's possession?* When we borrow a friend's tool or equipment, we take care to return it in good condition. We are aware that if we misuse or break it, we pay the price to replace it. Not so with this precious possession God has entrusted to us. No skill at my command can repair it once I break it. So why do I treat it as if I were its owner or creator?

In a Christian's life there is a higher authority and a diligent plaintiff: God and the conscience. We are free to ignore both, but the cost is high–temporally and spiritually. Even in these small daily excesses which are so easy to dismiss or overlook, others are hurt. Christ, who loves us as no other, would not have us confuse liberty and license. He is the first hurt and often the One left to pick up the pieces.

All I need to do is look around to confirm how deadly the eating and drinking sins are. The world is filled with people doing the same as I. I have a long list of kin and friends who ate, drank, or smoked themselves into a premature grave because "they liked it," "couldn't stop," or "didn't care."

The Bible is filled with illustrations, parables, admonitions, blessings, and cursing having to do with food use and misuse. Many of them applied to my own lack of discipline. It isn't that good choices aren't attainable. Often, however, I am too tired, too busy, or too rushed to make sure the right things are available.

It is *my* attitude about food that is important. I can enjoy any good thing, provided I choose and consume it without desecrating the temple–turning God's creation into something grotesque through excess and illness.

Fortunately God has given me fair warning by allowing me to see what happens to others who abuse food and the effects of abuse in my own body. I also have time to correct the habits I clearly see as out of God's perfect will for me.

God wants me to enjoy good things in moderation–and in the future, to reduce or eliminate that which I know is destructive. The good news is I don't have a food problem. If I did, I might wrestle with it for the rest of my life–as so many people on the *diet roller-coaster* do. What I must do is learn to obey God and *recognize that my disobedience is sin*.

I have found support. I pray for God's help in every decision and at every opportunity where I may be tempted to put my will before His.[40]

The Sin We do not Talk About

by LeRoy Dugan

Many years ago I found myself in one of the many taverns lining the streets of downtown Minneapolis. I was not there to get "smashed" but to evangelize. As some of you may have discovered, it is relatively easy to engage an inebriate in a conversation about God.

During the course of our brief dialog one of the men insisted that it was impossible for him to give up drinking. His redolent repartee moved me to a curt, convinced reply, "God can set you free from your slavery to drink!" I said it *firmly* because it seemed ridiculously easy for God to do such a small thing for one man.

When the interview had ended, I rejoined our witnessing group for the trip back home. We exchanged information concerning the various people we had met during the evening. Then I simply sat, looked out the window of the bus at the lights and dark silhouettes of the passing city, and thought about my new acquaintance. Somewhere between Franklin and 98th Street I looked down at my fingernails. And then it hit me! I was a nail-chewing addict! I had been nibbling away at my fingernails almost since infancy. I had attempted to break the habit many times, but had never really succeeded.

---

[40]*Pentecostal Evangel*, August 18, 1991.

Suddenly I realized how inconsistent I had been that very night. I had looked squarely in the face of a man fighting a monstrous habit of alcoholic addiction for years, flatly asserting that God could free him–and at the same moment I could not muster up enough faith to believe that God could cure me of a midget mania like nail-biting. It was an open and shut case of the pot calling the kettle black. One small addict trying to tell one big addict how to quit being an addict!

But "the sin we do not talk about" is neither drunkenness nor nail-chewing. It is something far more prevalent than either one, and much more "sanctified." It has several characteristics which set it apart from almost all other practices:

It can be carried on by people of all social levels. It can be done in public without creating the slightest scandal. It is frequently accompanied by prayer. It is as enjoyable to the old as to the young. It is always welcome where many lesser faults are not tolerated. It contributes to the untimely deaths of more Americans than any other vice, including alcoholism and the use of hard narcotics. It is one of the most popular and most widely accepted sins of modern Christians. It is called, in modern terms, *overeating*. In Scripture, it is more correctly labeled *gluttony*.

The sin we do not talk about. For many years I have pondered the matter, and wondered why there is such deafening silence on the subject which should command such attention.

It is only fair to say that many Christians do offer token resistance to this particular malpractice. They go on endless diets. They speak obliquely of their "weight problem." They veil their expressions of guilt with gentle humor.

But rarely does anyone call his sin by name and treat it as the crime the Bible says it is!

I am left with a logical dilemma. Let's put it in the form of a question: "How does one addict dare tell another addict he must cease his addiction?" To be more precise: How can a Christian tell an adulterer to stop his sex-addiction if he himself is still a "food-a-holic"? How can a believer challenge a sinner to repent of his sin if the believer himself has not repented of his food-addiction? How can a saint insist that a thief must stop stealing if he himself cannot refrain from over-eating? Why is it somehow more criminal that an appetite for drink or sex be uncontrolled than an appetite for food? Why is there more need for repentance of one sin than of another? By what biblical principle is overdrinking more heinous than overeating?

Does it not seem that one form of slavery is as bad as another? There would appear to be no essential difference between being bound by steel chains than by wrought iron. The high polish of the steel does not diminish the bondage one whit [bit]. Slavery to appetite is slavery to appetite. [It is slavery] whether it be the craving for sex, possessions, or food.

To cast the whole matter into the words of Scripture: "You are without excuse, every man of you who passes judgment, for in that you judge another, you condemn yourself ..." (Romans 2:1). Is he not actually telling us that we are in no position to help a slave until we ourselves are free?

We evangelicals say a great deal about "walking in the Spirit." And we should. We make much of the importance of maintaining a life in which the "flesh" is subservient to the Spirit. And we are correct in our emphasis. But let us be candid. Honest. Specific. The aspect of our humanity that screams the loudest for a place of dominance is none other than our appetite for FOOD. At *that* point the battle must be joined. At *that* frontier we must stop the invader!

There is not a person in the world who would want to face God with the admission that he had arrived in the next life a little early because he was shot attempting a holdup. Or was caught in a burning house of prostitution. Or had died from an overdose of heroin. Or had succumbed to bad liquor. Or had expired from cigarette-induced cancer.

Is there any person who would want to face that same God with the confession that his life had been cut shorter than necessary because he ATE himself to death? Does anybody really want to face the end result of caloric suicide? Certainly not.

But, more importantly, does any genuine Christian really want to be a bond servant to his own desire for food? Absolutely not!

Let me say here that I know there are exceptional people whose overweight has nothing to do with overeating. There are others who are thin although they overeat. Basically I am not talking about weight. I am talking about overeating. The Bible calls it gluttony and puts it in the same class as drunkenness.

None of us feels comfortable about overeating. We have tried to rationalize our way out from under the pressure of conviction, but deep within us we have known all along that it is wrong. Whatever we may have convinced our minds of, our consciences still needle us about our gluttony. We look in the mirrors at home and long to look trim and disciplined. We try all manner of things to conceal the physical results of our over-indulgence. We spend hard-earned cash in vain efforts to cancel out the evidence of our sin. And we do it all because we KNOW that it is wrong.

Might I suggest there may be ONE thing we have not yet tried? We have not dealt with this sin like we deal with other sins! As long as we only conceal it, we get no cure. As long as we label it falsely, we get no help from God. As long as we make it a joking matter instead of a moral matter, we will get no more divine assistance to overcome gluttony than we would to overcome bad temper, immorality, or drunkenness.

Let's start talking about the sin we do not talk about–not necessarily *with* each other; not *to* each other; but *to God*.

I am convinced that God wants to make Christians free from overeating just as much as He wants to make sinners free from drugs, drunkenness, and damnation.[41]

---

[41]*Message of the Cross*, Nov./Dec. 1974, pp. 13-15.

Section 7
Paul's Thorn in the Flesh

"There was given to me a thorn in the flesh ... For this thing I besought the Lord thrice, that it might depart from me. And he said unto me, My grace is sufficient for thee; for my strength is made perfect in weakness" (2 Corinthians 12:7-9).

A. **Paul's Thorn in the Flesh was ...** (Negative approach)
   1. Weak or diseased eyes, or
   2. Other forms of bodily sickness.

B. **Paul's Thorn in the Flesh was ...** (Positive aspect)
   1. A person or group of persons
   2. The fellowship of Christ's sufferings. ("If we suffer with Him, we shall also reign with Him.")

Was Paul's thorn in the flesh an oriental eye disease or other form of sickness which God was unwilling to heal? Aside from a purely academic approach, Paul's thorn might be defined as one of the biggest excuses for unbelief ever propagated by faithless preachers. By twisting the scripture slightly, and making certain associations, they conclude that God is not willing to heal the sick today because God was not willing to remove Paul's thorn.

Granted, if Paul's thorn was sickness, then we have no assurance it is God's will to heal anyone, for God is no respecter of persons. Then, we must either disregard the many scriptures which set forth the doctrine of divine healing for the sick, and disallow the many passages scattered throughout the Gospels which state that Christ (who came to do His Father's will) healed *everyone* who came to him-or charge God with discrimination against Paul. Evidently such a position is not wholly consistent with the scripture. Nevertheless, there is a positive Bible answer to this question which has plagued so many Christians. Perhaps the question can best be resolved by determining first what Paul's thorn in the flesh was **not**.

First, Paul's thorn was not weak or diseased eyes. True, Paul wrote to the Galatians, *"I bear you record that if it had been possible, ye would have plucked out your eyes and have given them to me"* (Galatians 4:15). Does this passage mean that Paul was afflicted with eye trouble? Such an approach is based upon mere assumption. The Galatians simply used a figure of speech expressing the extent of their love for Paul. Even today we hear expressions of commendation linked with such figures of speech as: "I'd give him the shirt off my back" or "I'd give my right arm to see him through this." Though we speak in these terms, we do not mean that our friend does not have a shirt to wear, or that his right arm is missing. We do not mean to be understood in that way any more than the Galatians meant to say that Paul's eyes were defective.

Yet some Bible interpreters strain the point even further by basing supposition upon assumption, supposing that Paul had a certain oriental eye disease called *ophthalmia* which caused extreme nearsightedness and profuse mattering of the eyes-a terrible malady. Support for this position is drawn from Galatians 6:11 where Paul wrote: *"Ye see how large a letter **I have written unto you with mine own hand.**"* This, they say, indicates Paul was so nearsighted-actually so near blind-he was forced to write using large letters upward to one inch in height!

First, consider the fact that we do not have one original manuscript written by Paul from which we can determine the size of the letters with which he wrote. Furthermore, not the word "letter" is singular, and *not* plural as would be necessary if it were to denote the various written characters of an alphabet. Paul was referring to the largeness of the epistle–the letter which he wrote-not the individual letters of the alphabet. According to *Strong's Concordance*, the word "large" speaks of "the quantitative form-how much." Paul then actually said, "Ye see **how much** I have written in this epistle with my own hand." (Some of Paul's letters were written by scribes as he dictated.) Paul showed his urgent concern f or the church at Galatia by communicating in his own handwriting.

Apart from the two passages considered here, there is no scriptural support for the idea that Paul's thorn in the flesh was an oriental eye disease. The fact is, Paul was divinely *healed* from blindness through the ministry of Ananias (Acts 9:18).

Now let's look at the scriptures that supposedly prove Paul's thorn was some form of sickness which made him extremely weak. To the Corinthians, Paul wrote, "I was with you in weakness ..." (1 Corinthians 2:3). His second epistle to the Corinthians reads, "I glory in my infirmities ..." (1 Corinthians 12:9).

At first thought, it would seem that Paul's infirmities were sicknesses, and that perhaps sickness was his thorn in the flesh. This position deserves our careful consideration. The word "infirmity" translated from the Greek [in Strong's Concordance], has two meanings: (1) weakness by reason of inherent, inborn frailty of the flesh; (2) weakness or impotency by reason of sickness. The scriptural setting leaves no doubt when the second meaning is intended. Luke 13:11-13 tells of a woman who was bound by an infirmity 18 years. Evidently some dread disease had left her muscles in a weakened condition, for she " ... was bowed together, and could in no wise lift up herself." Jesus said unto her, "Woman, thou art loosed from thine infirmity." The scripture clearly indicates when "infirmity" means weakness resulting from sickness. Otherwise, the first meaning is intended-the weakness by reason of inborn frailty of the flesh. Such was the case with Paul's infirmities.

Some picture Paul as a sickly, spindly man, but the Bible gives us to believe that he was a man of great vitality. There is no record of sickness incapacitating Paul for the work of the ministry, and his was a demanding ministry. Paul testified of God's grace, saying, "I am the least of the apostles ... but I labored more abundantly than they all." It is hardly reasonable to believe Paul was a sick man and still "labored more abundantly" than his fellow apostles who were well.

Paul's ministry demanded that he travel the then known world! Travel then was slow, strenuous, and often by foot. He ministered under the most adverse circumstances imaginable. Paul speaks reservedly of himself:

> "... in labours more abundant, in stripes above measure, in prisons more frequent, in deaths oft. Of the Jews five times received I forty stripes save one. Thrice was I beaten with rods, once was I stoned, thrice I suffered shipwreck, a night and a day I have been in the deep; In journeyings often, in perils of waters, in perils of robbers, in perils by mine own countrymen, in perils by the heathen, in perils in the city, in perils in the wilderness, in perils in the sea, in perils among false brethren; In weariness and painfulness, in watchings often, in hunger and thirst, in fastings often, in cold and nakedness. Beside those things that are without, that which cometh upon me daily, the care of all the churches" (2 Corinthians 11:23-28).

What a ministry! If that work were cut out for the strongest among us-doubtless that one would feel weak in the same sense that Paul felt weak. "Who is weak, and I am not weak?" Paul was no stronger than the other apostles. "If I must needs glory, I will glory of the things that concern mine infirmities [human limitations]" (2 Corinthians 11:29-30). No sick man could do the work that Paul did. It took all the strength of Paul and then additional strength from the Lord daily to maintain such a ministry-and therein was God glorified!

In his first letter to the Corinthians Paul readily acknowledged his human limitations in the face of a spiritual mission. He wrote:

> "And I, brethren, when I came to you, came not with excellency of speech or of wisdom, declaring unto you the testimony of God. For

I determined not to know any thing among you, save Jesus Christ, and him crucified. And I was with you in weakness, and in fear, and in much trembling. And my speech and my preaching was not with enticing words of man's wisdom, but in demonstration of the Spirit and of power:" (1 Corinthians 2:1-4).

The power of the Spirit stands out here in contrast above the weakness of the flesh. The words, "I was with you in weakness" do not imply sickness. In fact, the same Greek word translated "weakness" here is rendered "infirmities" in Romans 8:26: "Likewise the Spirit also helpeth our infirmities." It is also translated "infirmities" in Romans 8:26: "Likewise the Spirit also helpeth our infirmities." It is also translated "infirmities" in 2 Corinthians 12:9-10.

"... Most gladly therefore will I rather glory in my infirmities, that the power of Christ may rest upon me. Therefore I take pleasure in infirmities, in reproaches, in necessities, in persecutions, in distresses for Christ's sake: for when I am weak, then am I strong."

Paul was honored with a ministry of great power because he learned the truth of Christ's words: "Without me ye can do nothing." He realized the nothingness of himself, and his inability to do the work of Christ except in the power of Christ. Accordingly, he could say, "I can do all things through Christ which strengtheneth me" (Philippians 4:13). Paul's thorn in the flesh was only indirectly related to the infirmities in which he humbly gloried.

The Apostle himself plainly states what his thorn in the flesh was. "There was given unto me a thorn in the flesh, the messenger of Satan to buffet me ..." (2 Corinthians 12:7). The term "thorn in the flesh" can be best defined in the light of Bible usage. This figure of speech is used in four other places throughout the Bible: Numbers 33:55; Joshua 23:13; Judges 2:3; 8:7; and Ezekiel 28:24. None of these passages refers to sickness. They concern themselves with the tribes of Canaan which the Israelites had failed to completely drive out of the Promised Land. These idolatrous people were a continual source of trouble and were referred to as "thorns" in the flesh of the Israelites.

In like fashion, Satan used a block of unbelieving Jews to oppose Paul and the Gospel. These jealous religionists were a constant source of trouble wherever Paul went–from Jerusalem to Antioch, Iconium, Lystra, Thessalonica and back again. Paul referred to this opposition element as " ... *a thorn in the flesh, the messenger of Satan to buffet me."* By literal translation, to "buffet" means to "beat with many blows." Paul came against the unbelief of traditionalistic Jews with the Spirit and the Word, but they resisted him with physical force-actually beating Paul on occasion.

Evidently Paul was referring to such an occasion in 2 Corinthians 12:2-4 when he didn't know whether he was dead or alive. Significant to note, this incident took place 14 years before the letter was written, 60 AD, which brings us back to 46 AD. In that year, Paul preached the Gospel at Lystra, among other places, with miraculous results. While at Lystra, *"...there came certain Jews from Antioch and Iconium, who persuaded the people, and, having **stoned Paul**, drew him out of the city, supposing he had been dead"* (Acts 14:19).

Notice, certain "unbelieving Jews" stoned Paul, literally "buffeting" him with blow upon blow (the only time he was actually stoned). Such opposition from *his own countrymen* served to humble Paul lest he be *"...exalted above measure."* The unbelieving Jews definitely limited his success in the ministry. Paul had no power in himself to resist, and was often forced to flee the opposition. There remained but one resort. And, then the Lord, in His wisdom, did not promise to remove the thorny opposition, but simply said: *"my grace is sufficient for thee: for my strength is made perfect in weakness"* (Read 2 Corinthians 12:9-12).

Possibly Paul's humiliation was heightened by disfigured features resulting from much persecution. When Paul was stoned at Lystra, they dragged his unconscious form over the rough streets to a place outside the city. No doubt he suffered additional injuries in the process, for we can imagine that his persecutors were not too careful about the way they treated the body of their enemy "whom they supposed to be dead." At any rate, there must have been some lasting effects from the ordeal, for Paul wrote: "I *bear in my body the **marks*** [scars of service] of the Lord Jesus" (Galatians 6:17).

Jesus first suffered shame and insults at the hands of the *Jews* [before He was crucified]: *"They spit in his face, and buffeted him; and others smote him with the palms of their hands"* (Matthew 26:67). They plucked His beard; His visage was marred. ...

Paul knew intimately the fellowship of Christ's sufferings: the same Jews [through the Roman soldiers] that pressed a crown of thorns into Christ's brow became Paul's ***THORN IN THE FLESH***.

—Yvonne L. Davis

Bibliography

Blech, Rabbi Benjamin. *The Secret of Hebrew Words*. Northvale New Jersey, London, Jason Aronson, Inc., c1991 by Benjamin Blech.

Bragg, Paul C., N.D., Ph.D. *The Miracle of Fasting, Physical, Mental & Spiritual Rejuvenation*. Hot Springs, California, Health Science, n.d.

Brown, Arthur I. *God and You, Wonders of the Human Body*. Findlay, Ohio. Fundamental Truth, n.d.

Cohn, Joseph Hoffman. *I Have Loved Jacob*. New York, N.Y. American Board of Missions to the Jews, Inc. c1948 by Joseph Hoffman Cohn.

Cott, Allan, M.D. *Fasting: The Ultimate Diet*, New York, New York, Bantam Books, c 1975 by Jerome Agel.

Dake, Finis Jennings. *God's Plan For Man: Fifty-Two Lessons*. Atlanta, Georgia. Bible Research Foundation, Inc., c1949.

Flowers, S.L. *The Serpent's Fang*, Kansas City, Missouri, Beacon Hill Press, fourth printing, 1955.

Ginsburgh, Rabbi Yitzchak. *The Alef-Beit, Jewish Thought Revealed Through the Hebrew Letters*. Northvale, New Jersey, London, Jason Aronson, Inc., c1991.

Glazerson, M. *Sparks of the Holy Tongue*. Jerusalem, New York, Feldheim Publishers (first published 1975), c1975, 1981 by M. Glazerson.

Heidt, Henry J. *The Chosen People Question Box II*, Englewood Cliffs, New Jersey, American Board of Missions to the Jews, c1976.

LaHaye, *Transformed Temperaments*, Wheaton, Illinois, Tyndale House Publishers, c1971 by Tyndale House Publishers.

Lev, Mark. *Lectures on Messianic Prophecy*, 2nd Edition. Philadelphia, Pa. 1917.

McMillen, S.I., M.D. *None of These Diseases,* Old Tappan, New Jersey, Fleming H. Revell Company, c1963.

Munk, Rabbi Michael L. *The Wisdom in the Hebrew Alphabet*. Brooklyn, N.Y., Mesorah Publications Ltd., c1983.

Panin, Ivan. *The Writings of Ivan Panin*, New Haven, Connecticut, The Wilson H. Lee Company, c1918 by Ivan Panin.

Springer, Rebecca Ruter. *Intra Muros,* Elgin, Illinois, David C. Cook Publishing Co., c1898.

Wallis, Arthur. *God's Chosen Fast*, Fort Washington, Pennsylvania, Christian Literature Crusade, c1968 by Arthur Wallis.

General Index

A

abdominal, 125, 127
abdominal muscles, 125
Abel, 7, 48
Abiram, 102
abode, 95
Abraham Lincoln, 27
Absalom, 36
academic, 155
accomplice, 105
accosted, 132
accusations, 112, 148
accused, 132
aching, 103, 112
addiction, 148, 152
adultery, 9, 104, 106, 111
advertise, 32
Aescalapius, 86
aetoi, 50
afflicted, 155
aged, 95, 114
Aholiab, 38
alarm clock, 37
Aleph-Tav, 42, 43
allege, 32
allegiance, 141
almond-bowl, 80
Alphabet, 42, 43, 44
amazing, 13, 14, 35
American army, 123
Amman, 81
anah, 144
anchor, 61
ancients, 38
anesthesia, 3

angel, 120
angels, 19, 21, 29, 51, 70
anomaly, 123
anthropoid, 64
antidepressants, 129
Antioch, 158, 159
antithesis, 108
ants, 64
apathy, 10
Apocrypha, 8
apologetics, 4
apostasy, 4
apostate, 17
appendage, 26
aprons, 8
Arab, 81
Arabian proverb, 132
Arabic, 68
Archaeologists, 103
archaeology, 14
archaic, 11, 31
Architect, 84
architects, 38
Archives, 4
Aristotle, 11
arithmetic, 35, 78
Armageddon, 50, 51
aroma, 147
arrogance, 47
art galleries, 28
arthritis, 127, 129, 130
articulate, 115
artificial, 124, 131
Ascendings, 39
ascents, 39
ashamed, 54
Ashkelon, 103

asitos, 144
asparagus, 141
aspirations, 15
astonishment, 36
astronomical, 34
astronomy, 3
atonement, 97, 102, 159
attorneys, 4
aurora borealis, 33
authenticity, 14, 34
avarice, 66
avoirdupois, 36

B

babes, 28
baby, 80
Babylon, 40
Babylonian, 24
balances, 24, 56
baldheaded, 36
balloons, 125, 126
balm, 61, 104
bankruptcy, 92
banquet, 149
bar of God, 119, 120
Bashan, 69
bath, 45
battlefield, 51
beak, 9
beam, 113, 121
Beauty and the Beast, 24
bees, 64, 116, 133
beggar, 103
beggars, 29
behemoth, 33
belly laugh, 125, 126

belly-jiggling, 128
belly-shaking, 124
bellytime, 140
Belshazzar, 24
beneficial, 115
Bezaleel, 38
Bible Belt, 80
bibliomancy, 58
Bing-Bang Theory, 69
biologists, 18
biscuits, 141
bishop, 119
bishops, 7
bitter, 116, 119, 126, 139
blandishments, 26
blasphemy, 45, 120
blighted, 114
blind, 116, 156
blood pressure, 125
blood stream, 102
bloodstream, 125
blueprinting, 4
blues, 127
body mechanics, 149
bones, 49, 84
bonfire, 14
boogiemen, 8
bookkeeper, 54
boomerangs, 70
bored, 132
boredom, 148
bosom of God, 53
bossy, 67
botanical, 3
botany, 80
bouillon, 141
Brahmanism, 16
brain center, 114
brat, 49
breakfast, 137, 138
breeches, 8

Britishers, 32
bruit, 32
bubble soap, 125
bubbler, 107
Bulgarian, 68
bullet, 94
Burma, 23
burning bush, 73
burnout, 129
butterfly, 80
buttermilk, 141

C

Caduceus, 86
Cairo, 81
caloric suicide, 153
campus, 3
Canaan, 1, 22, 158
canary, 19
cancer, 130, 153
candid, 153
cannibalism, 108, 109, 110
canonizing, 35
canteen, 80
carcass, 50, 51
cardiovascular, 125
caricature, 61
carriers, 112
cartoon, 126
carved, 95
catalogue, 109
cathartic, 149
celery, 141
Chaldeans, 21
chamber, 149
chandeliers, 80
channeled, 92
Chapel, 3
Charity, 26, 27
Chebar, 73

checkbook, 54
cheerboard, 126
cheerful religion, 119
chemical, 18
chemist, 18
chemotherapy, 126
cheque, 59
chips, 28, 60
chiseled, 66
chloroform, 34
chocolate kisses, 126
cholesterol, 150
chortles, 128
chuckle, 124
chunks, 108
church history, 4
churn, 117
cigarette-induced, 153
circumstantial, 20
city-scapes, 126
Civil War, 27
climes, 12
clocktime, 140
clot, 91
clouts, 32
clown, 125
clucking, 54
coconut, 141
comedy video, 128
commentators, 41
compass, 30
compassionate, 103
condemn, 102, 109, 110, 116, 120, 153
condemned, 104, 105, 109, 119, 123
Confucianism, 17
congregation, 148
connotation, 70
consecrated, 102

conservatory, 28
consumed, 108, 109, 114
conveyances, 118
corn on the cob, 32
corpse, 50
correlations, 34
correspondence, 29
corrupt, 94
countenance, 85, 95, 111
counterpart, 44
Court of the Israelites, 39
Court of the Women, 39
Court of Women, 39
cowardice, 47
cranium, 9
creaking, 124
crocodile, 33
crucify, 64, 136
crusade, 121
crying, 130
crystal, 136
cults, 17
culture, 3
Culture Club, 11
cultured, 11
curds, 97
curse, 87, 88, 97, 99, 100, 115, 123
curse words, 99
cuticle, 32, 33
cynicism, 95

D

D-Zerta, 143
Damascus, 81
damn, 122
darku, 49

darn, 122
darnation, 122
date honey, 81
defiled, 94
degradation, 16
degrees, 39
demoralizes, 94
den of lions, 144
Department of Antiquities, 14
Department of Music, 3
desert mountain, 73
despondency, 95
detective, 71
deterioration, 129
deterrent, 147
devil, 21, 67
devils, 19, 27, 133
devouring, 108, 109, 110
diagnose, 99
dialects, 1, 12, 29
dialogue, 78
diaphragm, 126, 127
diaphragm muscles, 126
digestion, 101
disclaimer, 104
discord, 110, 111, 112
discrepancies, 11
discrimination, 155
diseased, 155
disembodied, 24
disfigured, 159
dishwashing, 137
Divination, 58
divine cosmetics, 4
divine currents, 91
divine silence, 117
divorce, 104
doctrine, 16, 50

dog fight, 109
doubletongued, 119
dragon, 33
dragons, 31
dramatics, 3
dream, 21
drunkenness, 105, 109, 152, 153, 154
dry goods, 5
dust, 18, 44
d'vash, 81
dynamo, 68
dynasty, 61
dyspepsia, 137

E

eagles, 22, 50, 51
earthquake, 6
Eastern, 37
Edom, 2
effervescence, 118
El Roi, 78
electricity, 34, 131
eloquence, 120
embryo, 3
embryology, 80
emotional drunkards, 37
emperors, 29
empires, 114
employer, 73
empty space, 34
emrods, 32
encampment, 132
engrave, 66
enriched, 92
entertainment, 144
entice, 21
entomology, 80
Epistles, 3, 29

erroneous, 117, 148
escapist, 149
Eshmoun, 103
etiquette, 4
euphemism, 122
evangelical, 80, 81
evil speaking, 101,
    102
evil spirit, 21
evolution, 13
exaggeration, 114
Example, 119
excavations, 103
execution, 18
exile, 39
expletive, 122
expositors, 41, 70
eye trouble, 155

F

factions, 109
fairminded, 16
fairy tales, 31
fairy-tale, 14
faked smile, 125
false witness, 110, 111
family peculiarity,
    122
family prayer, 137
family tree, 48
fathomlessness, 15
feathered arrow, 59
feeble, 150
fellow-workers, 113
ferret, 56
fevered brow, 61
fig leaves, 8
Final High Priest, 16
fingernails, 151
finite, 41
firmament, 43

first cousins, 48
fish, 6, 19, 43, 49,
    141, 142
flags, 54
flood, 50, 51
flower, 114
flowers, 32
folk wisdom, 25
folklore, 14
folly, 95
food-a-holic, 152
food-addiction, 152
forestalled, 119
fornication, 95, 106,
    109
fortress, 118
fount, 94
fountain, 118, 119
fowls, 51
foxes, 121
frailty, 156
fraud, 12
fretting, 91
frivolity, 115
frivolous, 119
frontier, 153
frown, 124
furnace of affliction,
    118
furnace of earth, 29

G

gabby, 118
Galilee, 21, 74
galley, 7
garden, 3, 6, 19
Garden of Eden, 6, 74
Gee, 122
gelotology, 125
genealogy, 48
Geneva, 7, 9

genius, 13, 15
Gershom, 26
ghoulish, 109
giant, 69
Gibraltar, 15
giggle, 124
giggling, 124
Gilead, 9
glands, 93, 127
glazed, 143
glittering peaks, 29
gnashed, 60
goad, 38
goals, 127
godliness, 64
gods, 7, 70, 71, 149
God's library, 84
Goethe, 12
goings up, 39
golden, 24
golden lampstand, 80
Goliath, 25
Golly, 122
Gomorrah, 20
goodwill, 95
gorging, 108
Gosh, 122
gosh, 122
Goshdarned, 122
gracious, 122
graduates, 3
graduating, 89, 90
grain, 32
grapple, 80
Great Unnamable, 6
Great Unspeakable, 6
grinning, 125
grudges, 92
guard, 93, 95, 114,
    116, 118
guffaw, 124
Guide Book, 15

guile, 120
guineas, 7
gulping, 108
Gutenberg Bible, 8

H

habits, 94, 95, 100,
    140, 143, 151
Haggadah, 80
hallelujahs, 124
Ham, 105
hammer, 61, 68
handwriting, 24
happy attacks, 124
hardihood, 16
harmony, 118
harp of David, 28
hasty, 115
hatred, 107, 111, 112
Hazak, 89, 90
headlines, 4
health-wrecking, 149
heartburn, 149
heinous, 152
hell, 19
helmet, 80
hemisphere, 59
heroin, 153
hieroglyphics, 72
hilarity, 124
hind, 33
Hinduism, 17
hippopotamus, 33
historical, 2, 20
holiness, 59, 64, 145
Hollandaise, 141
Holocaust, 72
Holy Hill, 106
holy men, 13, 29, 35
home-comers, 40
homosexuality, 104
honeyed tongue, 82

hormones, 129
horse, 33
horselaugh, 124
howling, 124
humiliation, 159
humility, 115, 118
humor, 125, 126, 128,
    129, 148, 152
humor therapy, 126
Hungarian, 68
hunger, 138, 141, 143,
    148
hypocrites, 112

I

icing, 26
Iconium, 158, 159
idle, 114, 115, 118,
    119, 120
idle words, 118, 119
idler, 119
idolatry, 101
ignoramus, 11
imaginable, 104, 157
Immanuel, 22
immigrant, 34
immorality, 101, 154
immortal, 106
immortality, 64
immune, 125, 128
impiety, 123
impostors, 12
impotency, 156
impunity, 109
impurity, 32
inappropriate, 27
incapacitating, 157
incessantly, 114
incongruous, 122
inconsistent, 152
index, 118

indigestion, 149
indomitable, 92
inebriate, 151
inebriates, 137
inexorable, 109
infancy, 151
infant church, 29
infirmities, 147, 156,
    157, 158
inflammatory, 129
information bureau, 76
inner jogging, 125
insatiable, 148
insinuating, 120
insinuation, 114
instrumental, 101
insult, 27
insurance, 73
intelligence, 15, 38
interjections, 122
interpolations, 8
interpretation, 21
interrupting, 66
intoxicated, 105
investigation, 34
invited, 27, 35
Iraq, 72
irradiate, 59
irrational, 11
irrefutable, 13
irreparable, 110
irreverence, 100
Ish Tam, 77
Islam, 81
Israeli Empire, 3
italics, 8

J

jackal, 33
jackals, 31
Japheth, 105
jaws, 105

jealousy, 91
Jethro, 72
Jewry, 72
Joab, 79
Job, 3, 7, 9, 24, 25,
    28, 31, 51
jokester, 76
Journalism, 3
Judas Iscariot, 27
judge, 113
justify, 105, 110, 116,
    121

K

kettle, 152
Key of Childbirth, 75
Key of Rain, 75
Key of the Revival of
    the Dead, 75
King Solomon, 118
King-size bed, 69
knights, 32
Korah, 102

L

labaneh, 97
languishing, 128
Lapidary, 80
lapidary, 4
lasciviousness, 109
late-onset diabetic,
    148
latticework, 59
Laugh Cure, 128
laughmobile, 129
lawlessness, 10
lays bricks, 73
Lazarus, 27, 103
leaves, 91, 141
legitimate, 117
Lenin, 24

leper, 100
leprosy, 101
leprous, 87, 101
Leshon Ha-Ra, 100
Leshon haKodesh,
    102
leukemia, 126
leviathan, 33
library, 8, 30, 61, 115
licensed, 109
lightning, 107, 116,
    133
lion, 121
lips, 107, 114, 116,
    118, 120, 122,
    123
lonely, 41, 61
long face, 119
loquacity, 117, 118
low-cal, 143
lust, 10, 66, 95, 109
lust of the flesh, 109
lustful, 137
Lystra, 158, 159

M

machinery, 68
magnifier, 8
make-believe, 37
malady, 132, 156
malevolent, 95
malice, 95, 96
malicious, 120
malignity, 91
malnourishment, 144
malpractice, 152
Malthus' law, 48
manuscript, 156
map, 30
marble, 66
march, 1

mark, 49, 66, 98, 107
marred, 112, 159
Martin Luther, 105
mashal, 38
Masoretes, 63
mathematically, 34
mathematics, 13
maxim, 38
meat, 32, 49
Medical, 3
medicine, 25, 86, 115,
    124, 125, 127,
    130, 149
Medicine Chest, 83
meditation, 38, 59,
    123
meek, 22, 46
melancholy, 119, 133
melee, 109
mellowed, 95
menace, 112
mercenary, 74
merry, 25, 26
Metanya, 69
metaphor, 25, 27, 43,
    82
mete, 106, 113
microbe, 95
microscope, 33
midget mania, 152
Midian, 25
midwife, 79
militate, 70
Millennium, 91
minced, 122, 123
ministers of reconcili-
    ation, 108
miraculous feat, 34
mirror, 30, 61
mob leader, 24
mobilization, 51
Mohammed, 68

Mohammedanism, 16
molehill, 116
molehills, 115
moneyed, 77
monkeys, 33
monologue, 78
monotheists, 70
moral, 106, 154
moral muscles, 37
mote, 113, 121
mountain goat, 33
mouse, 121
movie-goers, 37
multitudes, 112
Mumac Indians, 9
murder, 101, 104, 106, 107, 111
murmuring, 102
muscle, 114, 125
muscles, 127, 157
musician, 63
mystical, 26

N

Nabataens, 72
nagging, 124
nail-biting, 152
nail-chewing, 151, 152
naive, 92
naked, 105, 141
Naooktakumiksijik, 9
narcotics, 152
national pastime, 68
nearsightedness, 156
Nebuchadnezzar, 21
neighbor, 108, 121
neot kedumim, 96
nervous system, 93
nesteia, 144
nests, 96
neuroanatomist, 129

New Yorker cartoon, 148
newspaper, 59
nibbling, 151
Nimrod, 86
Nineveh, 2
Noah, 105
nonessential, 117
noose, 70
norm, 92
Nova Scotia, 9
numeric pattern, 13

O

obese, 142, 148
obesity, 142, 147, 148
obligation, 109
observatory, 3, 29
Occidentals, 48
Og, 69
ointment, 28
old-fashioned, 124
omnipotence, 18
omnipresent, 73
omniscience, 18
oncology, 129
One Mind, 35
ophthalmia, 156
opposition, 108, 158, 159
optimism, 126
orator, 75, 114, 115
organ, 28, 73, 101, 120
orgy, 109
Orient, 47, 48
Oriental, 48
oriental, 155, 156
orientalists, 72
ostracized, 28
outrage, 68

over-active fork, 142
over-eating, 96
overeating, 152, 153, 154
Owl, 110
oxdriver, 37
oxygen, 125, 131

P

pain, 86
painkillers, 129
palace, 29, 74
Palestine, 51
palm leaves, 8
pangs, 100
pantyhose, 142
parable, 9, 26, 27, 38
paragon, 64
paraphrase, 115
parental, 122
parroted, 10
passion, 95, 96
pastors, 2
patched, 32
pauper, 76
peacemakers, 9
peers, 92
perfunctory, 145
persecution, 159
Persia, 72
Pestilence, 132
petard, 27
Petra, 72
petty, 92
pew, 73
Pharao's, 72
Pharisees, 20, 145
phenomena, 13, 35
Philistines, 25
philosopher, 95, 114, 120

philosophy, 3, 15, 26
photography, 4
phrenologist, 71
physician, 85, 95
physics, 4
pick-up truck, 73
pickled, 124
pictograph, 42
piety, 95, 135
pilgrim, 61
pilot, 30
pious, 74
pita bread, 96
plastic, 94
Plato, 11, 12
platter, 32
Plautus, 112
plethora, 124
plucked, 155, 159
plurality, 70
poison, 91, 95, 102, 106, 115
poisoned, 86, 94
poisonous seed, 112
Polish, 68
polled, 32
polytheism, 70
popped, 49, 142
portals, 95
portico, 28
portly, 148
posea, 80
potential, 92
power plant, 68
prattling, 114
precepts, 38
precious stones, 80
precipitan, 19
prejudice, 10
prejudices, 92
preserved, 124
Preserver, 20

pride, 10, 95, 107
printing press, 8
prioritize, 127
prisonhole, 95
profanity, 123
professor, 119, 122, 125, 130
proliferation, 147
Promised Land, 87
propagate, 94
propagated, 155
prosper, 95
prostitution, 153
pseudo-scholarship, 10
psychologist, 11
Psychologists, 114
psychology, 4
ptoma, 50
publicize, 32
publisher, 115
Pulitzer Prize, 3
punsters, 61
pupil of the eye, 25
purifier, 80
purity, 64
pyramidical, 72
pyramids, 72

Q

quantitative, 156
quick, 18, 32

R

rabbinical, 69
railroad, 3
railway coaches, 5
Rainbow City, 72
rambling, 117
rapture, 50
rash, 115

rat, 60
rationalist, 34
ravine, 69
reagent, 18
reaps, 112
recital, 67
reconciliation, 108
recorded, 21, 59, 116, 118, 146
redolent, 151
reformatory, 121
refractory, 37
refrigerator, 141, 142, 148
refugee camp, 73
rehearsing, 67
religionists, 158
religious hangover, 37
remedy, 88, 102, 134
repartee, 151
resentment, 101
resh, 42
Resheph-Mukol, 103
reshith, 42
retaliate, 109
revealed, 18, 50, 54, 59
rheumatism, 125
riddle, 38
Rift, 72
Rip Van Winkles, 14
ritual fast, 145
Riyadh, 81
rock-crystal, 80
Romanian, 68
ROTCs, 3
rowing, 125
Ry-Krisp, 143

S

sacred, 16, 17, 45, 73
saddle, 32

saint, 67, 95, 114, 136, 152
saintliness, 64
salt, 28
salt water, 119
salutation, 89
sanctified, 102, 152
Satan, 19, 24, 27, 93, 112, 113, 158
sated, 150
satyrs, 32
Saviorhood, 59
scarlet thread, 79
scenario, 105
scissors, 115
scoundrel, 77
scourge, 132
screams, 121, 153
scribes, 20, 27, 45, 156
scrutinize, 56
scrutiny, 54
sea creatures, 43
self-centeredness, 96, 133
self-pity, 92, 133
seminar, 4
Septuagint, 39
serene, 95
serenity, 95
serpent, 86
servitude, 105
Seth, 48
severe, 105, 117, 130
sex-addiction, 152
sexual, 133, 144
shadow, 25
Shakespeare, 12
shallow, 121
Sharon, 28
shatter, 94
she-ass, 33

Sheba, 72
sheepfold, 73
Shem, 105
shoe, 114
shoes, 73
shovel, 14
shrinking, 64
sickly, 94, 157
silhouettes, 151
silver, 29, 140
Sin-Bearer, 16
Sinai, 3
Siq, 72
Sir Walter Scott, 5
skim milk, 117
slander, 100, 104, 105, 112, 113, 114
slavery, 151, 152
sleep, 128, 130, 133, 142, 144
sleeping draughts, 91
sloth, 66
slum, 114
smashed, 151
smeared, 121
smoke, 22, 26
snake, 86, 99
snicker, 124
snow, 5
snowball, 112
Sociology, 3
Socrates, 114
sod, 32
Sodom, 20
solder, 124
solitude, 61
Songs of the Steps, 39
sores, 91, 103
sour, 95, 124
sour face, 95
sovereign, 92
Soviet Union, 24

sows, 112
spades, 13
spasm/pain, 125
spasmodic, 127
speech center, 114
speedy, 32
sphinx, 72
spices, 29
spinal arthritis, 127
spindly, 157
spirituality, 12
sponge, 80
spontaneous, 124, 144
spoon, 115
Spurgeon, 17, 110, 115
stamina, 34
steeds, 32
steel chains, 153
stereophonic, 4
stimulant, 37
stings, 116
stolen, 105
stoned, 159
strands, 37
strata, 113
strawberries, 126
stress, 9, 56, 96, 119, 128, 129, 130
stripes, 97
suicide, 99
suma, 50
sunshine, 95, 116, 129
superfluous, 117
superscription, 63
suspicions, 112
swear, 100
sweet water, 119
sword, 61, 101, 113, 139
sympathy, 98, 104
synthesis, 109

T

Tabernacle of the Congregation, 101
tablets, 69
tackle, 127
Tale Makers, 112
talkative, 67, 118
talkativeness, 117
talley, 32
Tamar, 79
Tanna debe Eliyyahu, 73
Tattler, 112
tattler, 107, 112
taverns, 151
telescopes, 3, 29
temper, 95, 99, 100, 101, 141, 154
Tempter, 20
tensions, 124
tent, 105
test-tube, 18
thankful, 93
Theology, 4
theology, 80
Thessalonica, 158
thief, 105, 106, 152
thorny, 159
thunder, 6
tickle, 124
tickled, 37
tie, 115
tittle, 20, 30, 35
T'nach, 85
tolerance, 128
tolerate, 109
tornadoes, 33
tottering, 60
toys, 126

trade route, 72
traditionalistic, 158
train, 117
traitor, 99
tranquillity, 79, 91
transistors, 124
Translation, 51, 71
traveler, 29
tray, 32
tree of death, 87
Tree of Life, 19, 87
tribe, 132
tribes, 1, 158
trifles, 117
trinity, 70
tripartite, 84
trouble-shooting, 68
tsum, 144
tumors, 32
tunnel, 24
Tyndale Version, 7
tzu gezunt, 83

U

unbelief, 155, 158
unchristian, 99
unconscious, 159
ungloved, 118
ungodly, 50
unguarded, 121
unicorns, 31
unimpeachable, 18
university, 3
unruly, 101, 102, 115
unworshipful, 64
uplifting, 115
Upper Room, 53

V

vaccine, 3
variance, 95

vengeance, 96
ventilation, 125
Very Beginning, 42
vice, 121, 152
vinegar, 80
virgin, 22
virtues, 114
virtuous, 141
virus, 3
visage, 159
visionary, 74
vistas, 54
vitality, 91, 92, 157
vitamin C, 128
vomitarium, 149
Vulgate, 8, 63

W

wagging, 121
wedding feast, 27
welter, 114
West Point, 3
whispering, 110, 111
whit, 153
whoremonger, 106
wild ass, 33
wild ox, 31
willpower, 100
woodcut, 8
word-bloom, 117
wordiness, 117
worldliness, 115
worldlings, 137
wrath of God, 111, 112
wresting, 121
wrinkles, 95
wrought iron, 153

X

Xanthus, 120

Y

Yahweh Rapha, 83, 85
Yiddish, 68, 69, 83
yod, 20

Z

Zion, 5
Zippora, 72
Zipporah, 26
Zohar, 42, 74